**Rapid
Psychiatry**

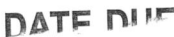

DATE DUE

RAPID PSYCHIATRY

Allison Hibbert
Alice Godwin
Frances Dear
All of
Royal Free and University College Medical School
University College London
London

EDITORIAL ADVISOR
Peter Raven

SERIES EDITOR
Amir H. Sam
Royal Free and University College Medical School
University College London
London

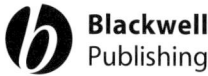

© 2004 A. Hibbert, A. Godwin, F. Dear and P. Raven
Published by Blackwell Publishing Ltd
Blackwell Publishing, Inc., 350 Main Street, Malden, Massachusetts
02148-5020, USA
Blackwell Publishing Ltd, 9600 Garsington Road, Oxford OX4 2DQ, UK
Blackwell Publishing Asia Pty Ltd, 550 Swanston Street, Carlton, Victoria
3053, Australia

First published 2004
4   2008

Library of Congress Cataloging-in-Publication Data

Hibbert, Allison.
  Rapid Psychiatry / Allison Hibbert, Alice Godwin, Frances Dear.
     p. ; cm. — (Rapid series)
  ISBN 978-1-4051-1324-3
  1. Brief psychotherapy—Handbooks, manuals, etc.
  [DNLM: 1. Mental Disorders—Handbooks. 2. Psychiatry—methods—
  Handbooks. WM 34 H624r 2004] I. Godwin, Alice. II. Dear, Frances.
  III. Title. IV. Series.

                                              RC480.55.H53 2004

ISBN 978-1-4051-1324-3

A catalogue record for this title is available from the British Library

Set in 7.5/9.5 pt Frutiger
by Kolam Information Services Pvt. Ltd, India
Printed and bound in Malaysia by Vivar Printing Sdn. Bhd.

Commissioning Editor: Vicki Noyes
Editorial Assistant: Nicola Ulyatt
Production Editor: Lorna Hind
Production Controller: Kate Charman

For further information on Blackwell Publishing, visit our website:
http://www.blackwellpublishing.com

Serious adverse effects of psychiatric drugs, 133
Treatment of psychiatric emergencies, 134

Appendices
Culture-specific disorders, 139
Eponymous syndromes, 140
Forensic psychiatry and the Mental Health Act, 143
Physical disorders with psychological consequences, 149

Glossary

We would like to thank our families and our friends at the Royal Free Hospital School of Medicine for their continued support.

We would especially like to thank Dr Raven for his encouragement, guidance and expertise.

July 2003
Royal Free Hospital, London, UK   A.H.
                                                                       A.G.
                                                                       F.D.

It has been a great privilege to be involved in the production of this innovative undergraduate textbook in psychiatry. When one of the students attached to my clinical firm first suggested the concept of a series of specialist textbooks written by students, for students, my reaction was a mixture of curiosity and scepticism. Luckily, a combination of Amir Sam's powers of persuasion and my curiosity overcame my scepticism. Together with Amir Sam, the authors of this book are among the very best students of psychiatry I have ever had the pleasure to teach. In the process of editing this book, I have learned a huge amount about teaching psychiatry, especially about the way that psychiatry as a subject is perceived by students. If you are a student thinking of buying this textbook, it has the great advantage that it presents the curriculum from the student's point of view. It pays particular attention to explaining those topics which students find especially difficult, without losing the emphasis on those conditions which clinicians consider to be important.

During the production of this book, I have seen the transformation of these authors from students to doctors. Needless to say, they used the drafts of this book to revise psychiatry for their final exams, and they all passed with flying colours!

I hope that you will learn as much from reading this book as we all did from producing it.

Peter Raven
January 2004

List of abbreviations

5-HT	5-Hydroxytryptamine (serotonin)	**CVA**	Cerebrovascular accident/Stroke
ABC	Airway, breathing, circulation (basic life support)	**CXR**	Chest X-ray
		DA	Dopamine
		DD	Differential disagnosis
ABG	Arterial blood gases	**DDAVP**	Synthetic ADH, used in childhood enuresis
ACE	Angiotensin-converting enzyme		
		DKA	Diabetic ketoacidosis
ACh	Acetylcholine	**DSM**	*Diagnostic and Statistical Manual* (US diagnostic guidelines)
ADD/H	Attention deficit disorder with or without hyperactivity		
		EBV	Epstein–Barr virus
ADH	Antidiuretic hormone	**ECG**	Electrocardiogram
ADL	Activities of daily living	**ECT**	Electroconvulsive therapy
A&E	Accident and emergency		
AN	Anorexia nervosa	**EE**	Expressed emotion
APP	Amyloid precursor protein	**EEG**	Electroencephalogram
		ESR	Erythrocyte sedimentation rate
ASW	Approved social worker		
		EtOH	Ethanol (alcohol)
ATP	Adenosine triphosphate	**FBC**	Full blood count
AUDIT	Alcohol Use Disorders Identification Test	**FFP**	Fresh frozen plasma
		GABA	Gamma-aminobutyric acid
B$_{12}$	Vitamin B$_{12}$		
BAD	Bipolar affective disorder	**GAD**	Generalised anxiety disorder
BMI	Body mass index	**GCS**	Glasgow Coma Scale
BN	Bulimia nervosa	**GHB**	Gamma-hydroxybutyrate
BNF	*British National Formulary*		
		GI	Gastrointestinal
BP	Blood pressure	**GP**	General practitioner
Ca	Calcium	**G-CSF**	Granulocyte-colony stimulating factor
CAT	Cognitive–analytical therapy		
		HIV	Human immunodeficiency virus
CBT	Cognitive–behavioural therapy		
		HR	Heart rate
CFS	Chronic fatigue syndrome	**HRT**	Hormone replacement therapy
CJD	Creutzfeldt–Jakob disease		
		ICD	*International Classification of Diseases* (WHO diagnostic guidelines)
CMHT	Community Mental Health Team		
CNS	Central nervous system		
CPA	Care Programme Approach	**ICP**	Intracranial pressure
		IgG	Immunoglobulin G
CPN	Community psychiatric nurse	**IGT**	Impaired glucose tolerance
		IM	Intramuscular
CPS	Crown Prosecution Service	**IQ**	Intelligence quotient
		INR	International normalised ratio (prothrombin ratio)
CRP	C-reactive protein		
CSF	Cerebrospinal fluid	**IPT**	Interpersonal therapy
CT	Computed tomography	**ITU**	Intensive Therapy Unit

IV	Intravenous	**PD**	Personality disorder
LFT	Liver function tests	**PMS**	Premenstrual syndrome
LP	Lumbar puncture	**PoM**	Prescription-only
LSD	Lysergic acid		medicine
	diethylamide	**PTSD**	Post-traumatic stress
MAOI	Monoamine oxidase		disorder
	inhibitor	**QT**	Q–T interval on an
MDMA	Methylenedioxy-		electrocardiogram
	methamphetamine (also		(ECG)
	known as Ecstasy)	**RIMA**	Reversible inhibitor of
MDT	Multi-disciplinary team		monoamine oxidase
ME	Myalgic	**RMO**	Responsible medical
	encephalomyelitis		officer
M/F	Male/female ratio	**RR**	Respiratory rate
MHA	Mental Health Act	**SAD**	Seasonal affective
	(1983)		disorder
MI	Myocardial infarction	**SHO**	Senior House Officer
MMR	Measles, mumps and	**SNRI**	Serotonin and
	rubella		noradrenaline reuptake
MMSE	Mini mental state		inhibitor
	examination	**SpR**	Specialist Registrar
MRI	Magnetic resonance	**(S)SRI**	(Selective) Serotonin
	imaging		reuptake inhibitor
MSE	Mental state	**SST**	Strange Situation Test
	examination	**STD**	Sexually transmitted
NA	Noradrenaline		disease
	(norepinephrine)	**SXR**	Skull X-ray
NHS	National Health Service	**TCA**	Tricyclic antidepressant
NMDA	N-methyl-D-aspartate	**TPHA**	*Treponema pallidum*
NMS	Neuroleptic malignant		haemagglutination
	syndrome		assay (test for syphilis)
NS	Nervous system	**TFT**	Thyroid function tests
NSAIDS	Non-steroidal anti-	**TIA**	Transient ischaemic
	inflammatory drugs		attack
OCD	Obsessive–compulsive	**U&E**	Urea and electrolytes
	disorder	**UTI**	Urinary tract infection
o.d.	Once daily	**VDRL**	Venereal diseases
OT	Occupational therapy		reference laboratory

Rapid series mnemonic

CONDITIONS

D:	Definition	Doctors
A:	Aetiology	Are
A/R:	Associations/Risk factors	Always
E:	Epidemiology	Emphasizing
H:	History	History-taking &
E:	Examination	Examining
P:	Pathology	Patients
I:	Investigations	In
M:	Management	Managing
C:	Complications	Clinical
P:	Prognosis	Problems

SECTION 1: PSYCHIATRIC HISTORY AND MENTAL STATE EXAMINATION

PSYCHIATRIC HISTORY
- Patient's personal details
- Reason for referral
- Presenting complaint
- History of presenting complaint
- Past psychiatric history
- Personal background
  Family history
  Personal history: childhood; school; occupations; relationships; psycho-sexual history; habits/dependencies; forensic history; present social situation
- Premorbid personality

MENTAL STATE EXAMINATION
- Appearance and behaviour
- Speech
- Mood
- Thought
- Perceptions
- Cognitions
- Insight

PSYCHIATRIC HISTORY AND MSE

Psychiatric history

PATIENT'S PERSONAL DETAILS
Name
Age
Gender
Marital status
Occupation
Religion/ethnic group

REASON FOR REFERRAL
- When was the patient admitted?
- Why was the patient admitted?
- Who was involved in admitting the patient, e.g. the GP, A&E, police, social worker?
- Is the patient in hospital voluntarily or detained under the MHA?

PRESENTING COMPLAINT
- Document this in the patient's own words.
- Document how long the patient has had the problem e.g. 'feeling low for the last few months'.

- Use open-ended questions to elicit these e.g. 'Can you tell me about the problems that brought you here?'

- Let the patient speak uninterrupted for the first few minutes before continuing questioning.

HISTORY OF PRESENTING COMPLAINT
- When did the problem start?
- Has it changed over time? If so how?
- Were there any precipitating events, e.g. bereavement, divorce?

Any other psychological symptoms, e.g. anxiety, guilt, suicidal ideation?
Any physical symptoms, e.g. disturbance of sleep or appetite, diurnal mood variation?
Any psychological/drug treatments for the current problem? If so, did they help?
Screen for any other problems. All patients should be asked about suicidal ideation, depression, obsessional behaviour and psychosis.
Any biological symptoms, e.g. sleep (initial insomnia, middle insomnia, early morning waking), appetite (up or down), diurnal variation in mood, energy, libido, concentration, tearfulness?

PAST PSYCHIATRIC HISTORY
- Any similar or other psychiatric problems in the past?
- Note GP visits, use of psychiatric services or any hospitalisations.
- Note when the problems occurred, for how long they lasted and the treatments received.

PERSONAL BACKGROUND
- A lengthy part of the psychiatric history that is divided into subsections.
- Approach this section by explaining to the patients that you would like to know more about them in order to understand their problems and to be able to help them better.

Family history
- Collect information about parents, siblings and other significant relatives.
- Enquire about age, occupation, social circumstances, any psychiatric disorders/other health problems, relationship with the patient.
- Make a genogram of the information.

Personal history
- Childhood: birth history (difficulties, prematurity); developmental milestones, delay in particular; description of early childhood; family and home atmosphere.
- School: leaving age; any truancy or school refusal, bullying; relationships with peers, teachers; exams taken and qualifications, further education.
- Occupations: list all jobs and duration of employment, reasons for leaving and any periods of unemployment.
- Relationships and psychosexual history: current relationship if any, are they sexually active, sexual orientation, any sexual difficulties, first sexual experience, any strange sexual experiences/abuse (NB: It is not appropriate to elicit disclosure of sexual abuse, but it may be volunteered by the patient), for women note age of menarche/menopause, past significant relationships – reasons they ended.
- Habits/dependencies: alcohol, tobacco and illegal drugs; record amount, e.g. units of alcohol per week; current and previous use; patterns of use; symptoms/signs of dependency and withdrawal; associated problems, e.g. problems at work.
- Forensic history: record all offences whether convicted or not (especially note violent crimes, sexual crimes and persistent offending).
- Present social situation: type of housing, who else is at home; financial circumstances including income, benefits, debts; social support – friends, relatives, social services.

PREMORBID PERSONALITY
- Difficult to assess in a short interview. Focus on consistent patterns of behaviour throughout life. This part should include an account from an informant, as no individuals can objectively describe their own personality. You must state which part is the patient's own description and which is the informant's. A useful starting question is 'How would you describe yourself when well?'
- Areas to include: attitudes to others in relationships; attitudes to self, e.g. likes oneself, confident; predominant mood, e.g. cheerful, optimistic; leisure activities and interests; reaction to stress, coping mechanisms.

Avoid reporting historical features in the mental state – it is supposed to be a snapshot of the patient at that time. The exception is when a previous feature of illness is no longer present, e.g. 'There was no evidence at interview of the persecutory beliefs which had been present on admission.'

APPEARANCE AND BEHAVIOUR

Dress, self-care: e.g. bright colours and make-up may be seen in mania, self-neglect in depression.

Behaviour during the interview: restlessness, tearfulness, eye contact, irritability, appropriateness, distractibility.

Psychomotor: poverty, stereotypes, rituals, other abnormal movements.

Rapport.

SPEECH

Rate (speed): slow/retarded, or pressured/uninterruptible.

Rhythm: normal, flattened or excessive intonation.

Volume: whisper, quiet, loud.

Content: excessive punning, clang association, monosyllabic, spontaneous or only in answer to questions.

Dysphasia.

Dysarthria.

MOOD

Observe the patients' mood during the interview and also ask how they are feeling:

(1) objectively (affect): your impression (appropriate/inappropriate) – depressed, elated, euthymic, blunted or flattened, anxious.

(2) subjectively: how the patient reports prevailing mood – depressed, elated.

NB: Can record biological features of depression here if not in the history.

Suicidal ideas? (See assessing suicide risk.)

THOUGHT

(1) Formal thought disorder (abnormal thought form):

The patient does not follow the usual constructions in communication and speech is less meaningful as a consequence. Common in schizophrenia.

- Derailment (Knight's move): there is a sudden intrusion of words from time to time, which in themselves would have been appropriate, but not in this context (the train of thought becomes derailed).
- Circumstantiality (loosening of associations): thoughts become vague and appear muddled.
- Thought blocking: the sensation of thoughts suddenly stopping.

(2) Abnormal thought tempo:

Acceleration (pressured thought, flight of ideas – may exist without pressure of speech) or retardation.

(3) Abnormal thought possession:
The patient experiences thought being controlled by an external agent – thought withdrawal, insertion, broadcasting (feeling that one's thoughts are being picked up by others).

(4) Abnormal thought content:
Preoccupations/overvalued ideas (these are strongly held and dominate and are not always illogical or culturally inappropriate).
Obsessions, compulsions, ruminations. Beck's cognitive triad – negative views of self, the world and the future.

Delusions
A delusion is a false belief, unshakeably held, which is outside the individual's normal social and cultural belief system.

Types of delusion:

- Grandiose – believe they have a special ability or mission.
- Poverty – believe they have been rendered penniless.
- Guilt – believe they have committed a crime and deserve punishment.
- Nihilistic – believe they are worthless or non-existent.
- Hypochondriacal – believe they have a physical illness.
- Persecutory – believe that people are conspiring against them.
- Reference – believe they are being referred to by magazines/television.
- Jealousy – believe their partner is being unfaithful despite lack of evidence.
- Amorous – believe another person is in love with them.
- Infestation – believe they are infested with insects or parasites.
- Passivity experiences – believe they are being made to do something, or to feel emotions, or are being controlled from the outside; somatic passivity – feel as though they are being moved from outside.

Delusions may be mood congruent, e.g. grandiose, persecutory in elated mood states; hypochondriacal, poverty-stricken, guilty, and nihilistic in depressed mood states.
See also the eponymous syndromes.
Delusions may also be classified as primary or secondary:

- Primary delusions arise 'out of the blue' without any identifiable precedent.
- Secondary delusions arise out of an underlying mood, psychotic phenomenon or defect in cognition and is understandable in the context. It arises out of an attempt to understand the primary morbid experience.

PERCEPTIONS
- Sensory distortions – increase in sound or colour sensitivity.
- Illusions – a misinterpretation of normal stimuli.
- Hallucinations – false perceptions in the absence of any stimulus; perceived to be coming from outside the person.

(1) Auditory: second-person voices directly addressing the patient (e.g. 'you are useless')

third-person – two or more voices discussing the patient (e.g. 'he's very powerful')

thought echo – voices echo thoughts before or after they happen

third-person commentary – voices comment on action (e.g. 'he's going out of the door now')

Ask about timing, triggers, number of voices, first or second person – e.g. the voice may be saying 'I am useless', 'you are useless' or 'he is useless'. Do they recognise the voice?

(2) Visual
(3) Olfactory: usually an unpleasant smell
(4) Gustatory: commonly a feeling that something tastes differently and this is interpreted as being the result of poisoning
(5) Somatic sensations: e.g. sensation of insects under skin or movement of joints

Hallucinations may be perceived by people when they are falling asleep (hypnagogic) or waking up (hypnapompic) – these are normal.

Pseudohallucinations are vague, lack clarity and recognised as coming from one's own mind.

COGNITIONS

Consciousness, orientation, concentration, attention, memory (see MMSE below).

Confabulation (inventing fictitious details about the past to hide poor memory).

Perseveration (excessive persistence at a task that prevents them from being able to turn their attention to something else).

Dysphasia, constructional apraxia, agnosia.

INSIGHT

How well the patients understand their condition.

Are the patients aware that anything is wrong?

What do they think is causing it?

Are they willing to accept help?

Formulation

- Summary – aim to give a very short precis of the relevant points of the case. Include the following: patient's demographic details, relevant background information, chronological presenting symptoms, relevant mental state findings.
- Differential diagnosis.
- Aetiology.

Consider biological, psychological and social issues.

Use the grid opposite to fit these together.

Factors	Biological	Psychological	Social
Predisposing (what made this problem likely?)			
Precipitating (why did you start then and not before?)			
Perpetuating (why is it still going on?)			

- Management plan including the following:

Short-term
need for history from other informants
physical: e.g. blood tests
psychological: e.g. neuropsychological tests
social: assessment of family situation or residence
need for observation by nurses
OT assessment
risk assessment

Long-term
psychological therapies
physical therapies
involvement of MDT

- Prognosis

Mini mental state examination

This test examines the patients' cognitive function. They are awarded a score out of 30. The scores available for each question are shown in brackets.

(1) Orientation: 'What is today's day? date? month? year? season?' (5) 'Where are we – country? county? city? hospital? ward/clinic?' (5)
(2) Memory (registration): 'I am going to name three objects. I want you to repeat them after me and then remember them, because I will ask you to name these objects in a few minutes – APPLE, BOOK, COAT'. Give one point for each one that they can repeat immediately. (3)
(3) Attention and concentration: 'Subtract 7 from 100. Keep subtracting 7 from each answer until I tell you to stop.' Maximum 5 answers. (5)
or
'Spell WORLD backwards.' Score 1 point for each correctly placed letter. (5)
(4) Memory (recall): Ask the patient to repeat the objects named above. (3)
(5) Language:

- Naming – Show the patient a pen and a watch, ask to name them. (2)
- Repetition – Ask the patient to repeat 'No ifs, ands or buts'. (1)
- Three-stage command – Ask the patient to take a piece of paper in the right hand, fold it in half and put it on the table. (3)
- Reading – Ask the patient to read and obey a command written on paper, e.g. 'Close your eyes'. (1)
- Writing – 'Write a sentence.' The sentence should have a verb and a subject. 'Go away' is not allowed! (1)
- Copying – Ask the patient to copy a design, e.g. intersecting pentagons. (1)

TOTAL /30

(1) Ask about current weight:

- What is your current weight?
- How often do you weigh yourself?
- What has your weight been in the past (highs and lows)?

(2) Establish their pattern of eating:

- Tell me about what you normally eat on a typical day, say yesterday.
- Are you dieting at the moment?
- Do you ever binge? What do you eat and what do you do afterwards? How do you feel during a binge?
- Do you think about food frequently (obsessional symptoms)?
- Do you eat out with friends?
- Do you like shopping/cooking?

(3) Enquire about additional methods of controlling weight:

- Have you ever used any methods of losing weight other than dieting?
- What exercise do you do?
- Have you tried slimming pills?
- Do you take laxatives/diuretics?
- Do you ever make yourself sick after eating?

(4) Physical problems associated with weight loss:

- When did your periods start, are they regular? Enquire about contraception.
- Do you think your libido is low?
- Do you feel tired and weak?
- Do you suffer from dizziness?

(5) Establish how they feel about their weight:

- What would your ideal weight be?
- Do you think you need to lose weight?
- What do you think about your body shape?
- If somebody said you needed to put on weight, how would that make you feel?

Alcohol history

SCREENING TOOLS

CAGE

The CAGE questionnaire is a screening tool to identify problem drinking. It is brief and non-confrontational, and so is a very useful bedside test. If 2 or more of the answers are positive, a full alcohol history must be taken.

C: Have you ever felt you wanted to cut down on your drinking?

A: Has anyone ever annoyed you by criticising your drinking?

G: Have you ever felt guilty about your drinking?

E: Have you ever had an 'eye-opener' (a drink first thing in the morning to avoid the symptoms of withdrawal)?

AUDIT

A more detailed screening questionnaire is the Alcohol Use Disorders Identification Test (AUDIT). This is a 10-item screening questionnaire with 3 questions on the amount and frequency of drinking, 3 questions on alcohol dependence, and 4 on the problems caused by drinking alcohol. This test is more complicated and must be conducted by a health professional trained in its use.

AUDIT questionnaire (scores in brackets by each question)
Please circle the answer which is most appropriate.

How often do you have a drink containing alcohol?
(0) never
(1) monthly or less
(2) 2–3 times a month
(3) 2–3 times a week
(4) 4 times or more a week

How many units of alcohol do you drink on a typical day when you are drinking?
(0) 0 or 1
(1) 2 to 4
(2) 5 or 6
(3) 7, 8 or 9
(4) 10 or more

How often do you have 6 or more units of alcohol on one occasion?
(0) 0 or 1 per year
(1) less than monthly
(2) monthly
(3) weekly
(4) daily or almost daily

How often during the last year have you found that you were not able to stop once you had started?
(0) never
(1) less than monthly
(2) monthly
(3) weekly
(4) daily or almost daily

How often during the last year have you failed to do what is normally expected of you because of drinking?
(0) never
(1) less than monthly
(2) monthly
(3) weekly
(4) daily or almost daily

How often during the last year have you needed a drink first thing in the morning to get yourself going after a heavy drinking session?
(0) never
(1) less than monthly
(2) monthly
(3) weekly
(4) daily or almost daily

How often over the last year have you felt guilt after drinking?
(0) never
(1) less than monthly
(2) monthly
(3) weekly
(4) daily or almost daily

How often over the last year have you been unable to remember what happened the night before because you had been drinking?
(0) never
(1) less than monthly
(2) monthly
(3) weekly
(4) daily or almost daily

Have you or someone else been injured as a result of your drinking?
(0) no
(2) yes, but not in the last year
(4) yes, during the last year

Has a relative, friend, doctor or another health worker been concerned about your drinking and suggested you should cut down?
(0) no
(2) yes, but not in the last year
(4) yes, during the last year

Scores > 8 indicate a likely alcohol use disorder.

FULL ALCOHOL HISTORY
Establish a drinking pattern and quantity consumed
- What is drunk (beer, wine, spirits, etc.)? Remember patients often underestimate this. It helps to go through a typical day adding up what was drunk and when.
- How much is drunk in units (e.g. if, they only drink vodka at home, ask how long a bottle lasts)?
- How much is spent on drinking?
- How often do they consume alcohol?
- Where are they drinking (home, pub, etc.)?
- At what time do they have their first drink of the day?
- Do they drink steadily or have periods of binge drinking?
- Is there anything that increases their consumption of alcohol (e.g. availability, stress, anxiety)?

Features of alcohol dependence syndrome
> 3 out of 7 for diagnosis of alcohol dependence syndrome (ICD guidelines).

(1) Stereotyped pattern of drinking
When and where do you normally drink? (You are looking for a lack of variety of situations where they drink, e.g. spends every evening in the same pub.)

(2) Primacy of drink
Is drinking alcohol important to you? Is it often the first thing that comes to your mind, e.g. when planning a social gathering?

(3) Compulsion to drink
Do you feel an urge to drink?

(4) Tolerance
Have you found that alcohol has less effect on you than in the past?

(5) Withdrawal
Do you ever feel shaky and anxious when you haven't had a drink, especially in the mornings?

(6) Relief drinking
Do you drink to get rid of these shaky and anxious feelings?

(7) Relapse after abstinence
Have you ever tried to give up/cut down on your drinking?
Did you seek help (e.g. AA, counsellors)?
What happened?

Establish risk factors and comorbid health problems relating to alcohol

Is there a family history of alcohol problems?

Are there any medical problems (e.g. dementia, neuropathy, liver disease)?

Are there any psychosocial problems (e.g. unemployment, relationship problems, depression and anxiety)?

Establish impact

Has drinking alcohol affected their physical or mental health?

Has drinking alcohol caused problems with relationships, work or the law (e.g. drink-driving, drunk and disorderly)?

Assessment of suicide risk

All patients being evaluated psychiatrically should be assessed for suicide risk. Never be afraid to ask about suicide – simply by asking you will not increase the likelihood of a patient committing suicide and remember that identifying a suicide risk can prevent a patient committing suicide.

Make sure the setting is calm, quiet and private. Establish a good rapport – use a calm, understanding and sympathetic approach.

Suicide risk is increased by a sense of hopelessness, the presence of psychiatric and medical illnesses, the presence of blatant and recurring suicidal thoughts, recent stressful events (e.g. loss of job or bereavement) and previous attempts at suicide. The risk is increased if the suicidal thoughts have led to formulating a plan as to how to go about it. A lack of social support also contributes to an increased risk, as does a lack of strong 'preventing' factors such as religious belief or children to look after.

These factors must be asked about in order to assess the patient's suicide risk. Below are some suggested questions that could be used for assessing suicide risk.

Eliciting a sense of hopelessness
- Do you still get pleasure out of life?
- How do you feel about the future?
- Does life seem worth living?
- Are you able to face each day?
- Do you ever wish you would not wake up?
- Do you find there are things to live for? Tell me about them.

Suicidal thoughts
- Have you ever thought of ending it all?
- Are you able to resist the thoughts?
- How do you feel about these thoughts?
- Have you ever thought about methods of suicide?
- Have you ever made any plans?
- Have you started to put these plans into action?

Previous attempts
- Have you ever tried anything before? Can you tell me about it?

Social support
- Have you ever told anyone before about how you feel?
- Do you have someone to confide in, close family or friends?
- Who do you live with – do you have company at home?

Identifying stressors that increase the risk
- Is there something in particular that is making you feel worse? Can you tell me about it?

Preventing factors
- What might prevent you from carrying out any plans?

Health problems
- Do you know if you are suffering from any mental health problems?
- Do you have any other health problems that are bothering you?

ASSESSING A PATIENT AFTER A SUICIDE ATTEMPT

The aim is to identify the risk of a repeat suicide attempt, the likelihood of this being increased by the presence of 'indicators of serious intent'. It is also important to explore any recent events/illnesses that contributed to the attempt.

Again use a similar approach as mentioned above for assessing suicide risk.

By questioning slowly and with graded questions, build up a picture to find out what led to the attempt, how it was carried out and how the patient feels.

Start with an open question around the event, e.g. 'Can you tell me about the day? Start from when you woke up in the morning, tell me how you were feeling and what happened. Take your time.'

INDICATORS OF SERIOUS INTENT

- A planned and premeditated attempt, well prepared for
  e.g. 'I have been collecting the packets of paracetamol for weeks; I have been buying a packet a week with my shopping; I knew that you needed quite a lot to kill yourself and most shops will only sell one packet at a time'

- Attempt carried out in isolation, i.e. precautions taken to avoid interventions
  e.g. 'I locked my door so no one could get in'

- Attempt timed to minimise risk of discovery
  e.g. 'I waited until my flatmates went away so no one would find me'

- Suicide attempt communicated prior to attempt
  e.g. 'I had discussed with my friend that I felt suicidal'

- Final acts in anticipation of death
  e.g. 'I had written suicide notes and posted them to all my friends and family'

- Violent, active methods, or quantities of drugs used that were known to be lethal
  e.g. 'I knew that if I tried to cut the veins in my neck, it would be more effective than slitting my wrists'

- Person thought the act would be final and irreversible
  e.g. 'I thought that I would bleed to death if I cut my wrists'

- Person states that the aim was to kill self
  e.g. 'I wanted to die, I don't want to suffer like this anymore'

- Person regrets surviving the attempt
  e.g. 'I am angry with my flatmate for calling the ambulance'

- Numerous previous attempts
  e.g. 'This is the third time I have tried to kill myself; I am a failure, I can't even do that right!'

SECTION 2: DIFFERENTIAL DIAGNOSIS

SYMPTOMS
Emotions: tension, irritability.
Cognitions: exaggerated fears, worries.
Behaviour: avoidance of feared situation, checking, seeking reassurance.
Somatic: tight chest, hyperventilation, palpitations, decreased appetite, nausea, tremor, aches and pains, insomnia, frequent desire to pass urine and stools.

DIFFERENTIAL DIAGNOSIS
Psychiatric
GAD
Panic disorder (see below)
Phobias
OCD
PTSD
Acute stress disorder
Depression
Substance misuse – especially withdrawal symptoms
PD
Dementia

Medical
Hypoglycaemia
Hyperthyroidism
Phaeochromocytoma
Delirium

MANAGEMENT
Full history and MSE.
Exclude medical disorders – glucose, TFT, etc.
Acute anxiety may be relieved by anxiolytics, e.g. benzodiazepines, but for short courses only. Patients may become dependent on them if used long term.
Antidepressants may help anxiety, even when the patient is not depressed.
Try to find out the cause/precipitants of anxiety – treat with psychological therapy, e.g. CBT.

The depressed patient

SYMPTOMS

Main features: persistent low mood, anhedonia, lack of energy, decreased
  concentration and attention, bleak and pessimistic views of future, feelings
  of guilt or worthlessness, ideas of self-harm or suicide.
Somatic features: sleep disturbance, decreased appetite, weight loss,
  constipation, amenorrhoea, decreased libido, diurnal variation of mood.

DIFFERENTIAL DIAGNOSIS

Psychiatric

Depression
BAD
Anxiety
PTSD
Schizophrenia
Schizoaffective disorder
Dementia
Substance misuse (chronic alcohol)
Borderline personality disorder

Medical

Hypothyroidism
Cushing's syndrome
Hypercalcaemia (malignancy)
Infections (HIV, syphilis)
Multiple sclerosis
Parkinson's disease
Medication (sedatives, anticonvulsants, steroids)

Others

Life events involving loss (e.g. death of partner)

MANAGEMENT

Full psychiatric evaluation and assess for suicidal ideation and psychotic
  features.
Exclude medical cause for depression.
Antidepressants.
Psychological therapies.

SYMPTOMS

Main features: elevation of mood, overactivity, overcheerfulness, overtalkativeness.

Other features: irritability, flight of ideas, distractibility, grandiose ideas, decreased sleep, delusions (mood-congruent), hallucinations, impaired judgement, irresponsibility, loss of normal social inhibitions, promiscuity, decreased appetite.

DIFFERENTIAL DIAGNOSIS

Psychiatric

Hypomania
Mania
Mania with psychosis
Schizoaffective disorder
Schizophrenia
Substance misuse (cocaine, amphetamines), acute intoxication, drug-induced psychosis
Brief reactive psychosis (to stressful situation)

Medical

Brain disorders affecting the frontal lobes (e.g. space-occupying lesion, HIV infection, syphilis, Alzheimer's disease)
Alcohol withdrawal
Corticosteroids
Anabolic androgenic steroids
Hyperthyroidism

MANAGEMENT

During the interview maintain a calm, non-confrontational manner. Manic patients may become aggressive or violent in response to even minor irritations. Antipsychotics may be used in the acute phase (see Bipolar Disorder for more information).

Admit if overt mania.

Exclude other/medical causes.

Antipsychotics in acute episode (e.g haloperidol).

Lithium is used as prophylaxis for recurrent mania (BAD).

ECT in severe cases resistant to other treatment.

SYMPTOMS

Features: auditory, visual, somatic, olfactory or gustatory hallucinations. Auditory and somatic are more likely in psychiatric disorders, while visual and olfactory suggest an organic disorder.

DIFFERENTIAL DIAGNOSIS

Psychiatric

Schizophrenia
Schizoaffective disorder
Mania with psychosis
Severe depression with psychosis
Alcohol and drug misuse, e.g. hallucinogenic drugs – LSD, 'magic mushrooms'
Delirium tremens (medical emergency)/acute alcohol intoxication

Medical

Epilepsy, e.g. temporal lobe
Space-occupying lesion
Delirium
Metabolic disturbances, e.g. liver failure
Infection – encephalitis
Head injury

MANAGEMENT

Full psychiatric assessment.
Exclude organic disorders.
Antipsychotic drugs for psychosis.
Antipsychotic drugs may take 10–14 days to have effect, but cause sedation in the meantime. The patient will require admission and monitoring.

A discrete episode of extremely severe anxiety, which may occur in many of the anxiety disorders. If the panic attacks are recurrent and cannot be explained by other psychological or physical illness, panic disorder is diagnosed. The circumstances of the attack need to be clarified to exclude other disorders.

In a panic attack, the anxiety starts abruptly in the absence of any objective danger and reaches a peak within a few minutes. The anxiety is very intense, but has a limited duration (usually 10–40 minutes).

SYMPTOMS
Autonomic
Palpitations/chest pain
Sweating
Trembling/numbness/tingling
Dry mouth/nausea
Muscle tension
Chills/hot flushes
Dizziness

Behavioural
Urge to get away from the current situation (flight)
Restlessness

Cognitive
Perception of difficulty in breathing/choking sensation
Unpleasant feeling of anticipation/threat
Fear of losing control, dying
Derealisation/depersonalisation

DISORDERS THAT FEATURE PANIC ATTACKS
Specific phobia
Agoraphobia
Social phobia
GAD
Panic disorder
OCD

The patient with obsessions/compulsions

DIFFERENTIAL DIAGNOSIS

SYMPTOMS

Unwanted distressing thoughts/images entering the patient's mind even though they try to resist them (obsessions). Thoughts are recognised as the patients' own.

The patients may feel they must perform stereotyped acts to ease their anxiety (compulsion). May be repetitive and recognised as senseless.

DIFFERENTIAL DIAGNOSIS

OCD
Anankastic personality disorder
Depression
Psychosis, e.g. schizophrenia
AN
Phobic disorders
Gilles de la Tourette's syndrome/tic disorders

MANAGEMENT

Full history and MSE.

In particular find out about any features of depression (it accounts for up to 30% of obsessional symptoms). Have they always been perfectionist-type of persons?

Are they having any other symptoms that might suggest psychosis: thought insertion, withdrawal, broadcast, hallucinations?

Treat OCD with CBT, although SRIs may reduce symptoms.

Treat depression – SRIs.

SYMPTOMS

Underweight patient: BMI < 19. The patient may complain of amenorrhoea, constipation, cold intolerance, fatigue, irritability.

DIFFERENTIAL DIAGNOSIS

Psychiatric

AN
BN – these patients are more likely to have normal BMI
Depression/hypomania/mania
Psychosis/schizophrenia
OCD

Medical

Any disorder causing weight loss, especially:

- malignancy
- thyrotoxicosis
- inflammatory bowel disease

MANAGEMENT

Full history and MSE. Diet history. Has there been any deliberate weight loss, excessive exercise, restriction dieting, vomiting or laxative abuse? (Suggests AN or BN.)

Are there any features of depression or psychosis?

Are there any other symptoms?

Exclude medical cause for weight loss – TFT, investigate any other symptoms. Malignancy must be excluded.

Aim to increase BMI to normal range (20–25). Inpatient treatment may be needed if weight < 65% of normal or if suicide risk.

The patient who overeats

SYMPTOMS
Bingeing food, then vomiting/purging with laxatives. Preoccupation with body weight and shape.

DIFFERENTIAL DIAGNOSIS
Psychiatric
BN
Atypical depression/SAD
PD

Medical
Kleine–Levin syndrome
Klüver–Bucy syndrome

MANAGEMENT
Full history and MSE. Features of depression? In SAD, patients may have increased appetite. Antidepressants may have an antibulimic effect. Medical stabilisation. Establish normal eating pattern.

SYMPTOMS
Alert with eye movements only/absent body movements.
Mutism (absent speech).
Absent movements.
Decreased attention span for environmental stimuli.
Speech may be present but there may be amnesia for personal identity
    and history.

DIFFERENTIAL DIAGNOSIS
Psychiatric
Schizophrenia (catatonic state)
Affective psychosis (depressive stupor)
Neuroleptic malignant syndrome
Psychogenic amnesia
Conversion disorder

Medical
Hypoglycaemia
Delirium
Encephalitis
Parkinson's disease
CVA
Acute intoxication, e.g. alcohol, solvents, phencyclidine

MANAGEMENT
ABC.
Exclude life-threatening brain pathology.
Check vital observations – BP, pulse, GCS.
Initially obtain brief history from an informant (? known psychiatric illness,
    medication, illicit substances; is the patient deaf and/or blind? what
    language does the patient speak?).
Perform complete physical examination.
Perform investigations guided by the history and examination.
Ensure that the patient is adequately hydrated – IV fluids.
Once life-threatening brain injury has been excluded, obtain a full history from
    an informant, obtain old notes and attempt MSE on the patient.
Admit the patient; further management will depend on the underlying
    aetiology.

SECTION 3: ADULT PSYCHIATRIC DISORDERS

At any one time, 20% of the adult population in the UK has a psychiatric illness. Only a very small proportion of these are psychiatric inpatients. The majority are cared for in the community. The patient may present to their GP, outpatient clinics, A&E departments, medical or surgical wards, or even end up in the care of the police service. Approximately 25% of GP consultations are for psychiatric illnesses.

As people now live longer, the proportion of the population who are over 65 years is increasing. Illnesses of all sorts are more common in older people. It is important to realise that *most old people are not demented*. However, dementing illnesses do become more common with increasing age.

There are some normal psychological changes that accompany the ageing process. Older people are usually not involved in as wide a range of activities as younger people. This may be due to poor health, income, retirement or reduced drive and ambition. Their acquisition of new skills and response to new situations is not so good as it used to be.

A lot of older people live alone, either in houses which may be too large for them to maintain, or in sheltered accommodation which may be cramped and impersonal.

Retirement may be a very stressful experience. There is a loss of income, routine, challenges, company and status. There are likely to be further losses, such as bereavements, and loss of health and fitness with increasing age.

Psychiatric illnesses in old age are often closely related to physical illnesses and disability, or their medical treatments.

There are, therefore, many stresses in ageing which may provoke psychiatric illness. However, whether or not persons develop a psychiatric illness as a result of these stresses will depend on their premorbid personality traits, coping strategies and support.

THE GERIATRIC DEPRESSION QUESTIONNAIRE

This is a useful tool for assessing mood disorders in the elderly. Depression is very common in the elderly, and they may not realise themselves that they are depressed.

Score 1 for the underlined Yes/No answers. Score > 5 suggests depression.

Please answer all the following questions 'yes' or 'no'.

(1)	Are you basically satisfied with your life?	Yes/<u>No</u>
(2)	Have you dropped many of your activities and interests?	<u>Yes</u>/No
(3)	Do you feel that your life is empty?	<u>Yes</u>/No
(4)	Do you often get bored?	<u>Yes</u>/No
(5)	Are you in good spirits most of the time?	Yes/<u>No</u>
(6)	Are you afraid that something bad is going to happen to you?	<u>Yes</u>/No
(7)	Do you feel happy most of the time?	Yes/<u>No</u>
(8)	Do you often feel helpless?	<u>Yes</u>/No
(9)	Do you prefer to stay home, rather than going out and doing new things?	<u>Yes</u>/No
(10)	Do you feel you have more problems with memory than most?	<u>Yes</u>/No
(11)	Do you think it is wonderful to be alive now?	Yes/<u>No</u>
(12)	Do you feel pretty worthless the way you are now?	<u>Yes</u>/No
(13)	Do you feel full of energy?	Yes/<u>No</u>
(14)	Do you feel that your situation is hopeless?	<u>Yes</u>/No
(15)	Do you often think that most people are better off than you?	<u>Yes</u>/No

'Normal' grief reaction following the death of a spouse/close relative may last for up to 2 years. It is often characterised firstly by shock and disbelief, then sometimes feelings of anger, guilt and self-blame. Later they may 'pine' for the relative, feel despair and sadness and have pseudohallucinations that the person is talking to them. Finally there is acceptance. Abnormal grief is a stress reaction.

D: 'Abnormal grief' – delayed onset, higher intensity symptoms. The patient may stay at one stage of the grieving process for a long time (shock, disbelief, denial) so that grief is prolonged.

A: Unknown.

A/R: Sudden/unexpected death, problems in the relationship resulting in ambivalence to the bereavement, or being unable to grieve due to 'putting on a brave face' for others (e.g. children).

E: Normal.

H: May have a history of difficult relationship with the deceased (e.g. stormy or overinvolved). Delayed onset of grief. Symptoms such as shock, disbelief, anger, sadness and despair may be severe. May feel depressed or have suicidal thoughts (especially related to a desire to be with the deceased).

E: MSE
A&B: May show appearance of self-neglect.
S: Slow, distracted.
M: Low.
T: Suicidal ideas.
C: Impaired concentration.
I: Good.

I: None specifically.

M: Bereavement counselling, CBT.
Antidepressants.
Monitor suicide risk.

C: Depression.
Substance misuse.
Suicide.

P: May respond to CBT. Grief reactions should wane with time.

Acute stress disorders

ADULT PSYCHIATRIC DISORDERS

D: Sudden onset (within hours) emotional response to a severe stress (such as being attacked). Begins and ends within hours to days of the event.

A: Broad range of stressors of overwhelming importance, e.g. physical/ sexual assault, major road traffic accident, war.

A/R: May represent a maladaptive response to stress. There may be a higher incidence in anxious or neurotic patients.

E: Unknown. There is an exaggerated response to the severe stress. May occur in any previously well person under extreme circumstances.

H: Severe stressor, e.g. attack, accident. Feelings of intense anxiety, accompanied by sweating, palpitations, dry mouth, vomiting. Patient may feel dazed with 'nervous shock'. May have amnesia of the event or denial. Reduced sleep/nightmares.

E: Autonomic arousal – tachycardia, hypertension, sweating.
MSE
A&B: Anxious, restless, may wander aimlessly or be hyperactive.
S: May be confused.
M: Fearful, low mood.
T: Amnesia/denial.
C: Amnesia. Otherwise normal.
I: Good.

I: Exclude other neuroses, psychoses or organic disorders producing delirium. CT head to exclude rising ICP if there is any history of head injury.

M: Remove the stressor if possible. Reassurance. The patient should try to recall the events. Short-term anxiolytics (e.g. benzodiazepines) may aid sleep and help relieve symptoms.

C: May progress to PTSD.

P: Symptoms should abate within a few days. If they persist, this suggests the patient is at risk of developing PTSD.

D: Prolonged severe abnormal response to stress beginning within 1 month of a stressful life event, e.g. divorce, and lasting no longer than 6 months.

A: Life events, e.g. moving house, divorce, being made redundant.
Abnormal psychological responses to stressful life events.

A/R: May be more likely in patients with poor coping skills, e.g. those with fearful/anxious PDs.

E: Normal.

H: Following a life event. The patient has symptoms of anxiety and depression but not severe enough to diagnose anxiety/depressive disorder.
Symptoms of anxiety – irritability, increased arousal, insomnia.
Symptoms of depression – tearfulness, low mood. But usually no biological features of depression (i.e. decreased sleep and appetite).
Adjustment to a terminal illness may follow a similar course to bereavement – shock and denial, anger, sadness and finally acceptance.

E: Anxiety. May have increased autonomic arousal (i.e. increased BP and pulse rate).
MSE
A&B: Fearful, anxious, sweating, tremor.
S: Normal.
M: Low, depressed.
T: Preoccupation with the event.
C: Poor concentration.
I: Poor.

I: None specifically.

M: Remove stressor if possible. Supportive psychotherapy, teaching about coping mechanisms and problem-solving techniques.

C: Short-term disruption of work and social life.

P: Usually improve following resolution of the cause.

ADULT PSYCHIATRIC DISORDERS

D: Anxiety when in places/situations from which escape may be difficult/embarrassing, e.g. crowds, open spaces. Fear of having panic attacks/fainting in such situations.

A: Exact unknown. There is increased incidence of life events immediately prior to onset.

A/R: Dependent personality traits.
Other anxiety disorders.
Panic disorder.

E: 60% of all phobic disorders seen by specialists.
F > M.
Age of onset 15–35 years, earlier in those with childhood separation anxiety.

H: Consistent and marked fear reported, or avoidance of
- crowds
- public places
- travelling alone
- travelling away from home

These situations promote anxiety.

Physical
palpitations
sweating
trembling
nausea
chest tightness
choking/shortness of breath

Cognitive
feeling dizzy
fear of dying
fear of going crazy
derealisation/depersonalisation

Avoidance behaviour, or may require a companion to go to a busy place.

E: Normal unless in that situation. May have anticipation anxiety. Condition may be severe and the person housebound. May have a panic attack if exposed.

I: None specifically.

M: Exposure therapy, gradually increasing, e.g. walking increasing distances from home each day. CBT.

C: Isolation, self-neglect.
Secondary depression.

P: Course fluctuating. If it lasts > 1 year, it will be unchanged at 5 years if untreated.

D: Eating disorder characterised by refusal to maintain adequate body weight (BMI < 17.5), distorted body image, intense fear of fatness and amenorrhoea (at least 3 cycles).

A: Exact unknown.

Biological
genetic (monozygotic > dizygotic concordance 60 : 10; increased risk if family history)
dysfunction of 5-HT neurotransmitter system

Psychosocial
sociocultural view that thinness is attractive
family relationships, e.g. overinvolved parents
personality, e.g. perfectionism, low self-esteem

A/R: Social
Western society
certain occupations, e.g. ballet, modelling, high-achieving schools
premorbid obesity

E: Prevalence: 1–2% in girls aged 12–18 years; 95% are female.
Average age of onset: girls 13–20 years; boys 17–24 years.

H: Biological
fatigue
amenorrhoea
constipation
cold intolerance

Behavioural
excessive exercise
restriction dieting
vomiting
laxative and diuretic abuse

Psychological
distorted perception of weight
dread of gaining weight/fatness
depression/anxiety/OCD
social isolation

E: Physical
gaunt and emaciated
dehydrated
muscle weakness
cold extremities
bradycardia and hypotension
fine lanugo hair

MSE
A&B: Thin, weak, slow.
S: Slow, slurred.
M: Low.
T: Preoccupation with food; overvalued ideas about weight and appearance.
P: Rarely, re-feeding psychosis.
C: Poor.
I: Often poor.

I: Blood: FBC, U&E, LFT, amylase, lipids, glucose, endocrinological investigations.

M: (1) Aim to increase weight to BMI 20–25.
(2) Hospitalise if very low weight/suicide risk.
(3) Monitor muscle power, BP, biochemistry, weight.
(4) Psychotherapies: family, CBT.
(5) Drug treatments: antidepressants, nutritional feeds. Metoclopramide to increase gastric emptying and reduce bloating.

C: Osteoporosis, metabolic/endocrine disturbance, arrhythmias, renal/liver/pancreatic damage, suicide.

P: Variable: mortality up to 20% (from cardiac causes/suicide), recovery up to 33%.

D: Also known as manic depression. Involves recurrent episodes of both depression and mania. During episodes there is significant disturbance of the patient's mood and activity levels. The recovery between episodes is usually complete and the frequency and pattern of episodes is variable.

A: **Genetic:** These factors have a strong contribution to BAD. Monozygotic twins have a 68% chance of concordance. Increased risk × 5 in those people who have a first-degree relative with BAD.

Precipitants: Life events (e.g. exams, end of relationship, pregnancy, death of loved one) may act as triggers for BAD relapse.

A/R: Incidence higher in social classes I and II and in urban areas. Increased risk of manic episodes in early post-partum period. Relapse rate is high especially if the first episode is in adolescence or early adult life.

E: Lifetime risk 1%. M/F = 1 : 1.

First episode usually during twenties and more commonly mania.

H: Hypomania – persistent mild elevation of mood (> 3 days) with increased activity and energy, decreased sleep, increased irritability, decreased concentration but increased planning and new ventures. The overactivity is poorly directed so that little is accomplished. Mild overspending. Overfamiliarity and increased libido.

Mania without psychotic symptoms – as above but to a greater extent. > 1-week duration with complete disruption of work and social life. Feelings of high creativity and mental efficiency can lead to grandiose ideas. Expenditure can be excessive and lead to debts. Loss of normal social inhibitions can lead to sexual disinhibition. Reduced sleep may lead to physical exhaustion. Extremes of appetite. Heightened sensory awareness.

Mania with psychotic symptoms – as above. Grandiose or persecutory delusions and auditory hallucinations may be present and are often mood congruent. Aggressive acts.

Depression – see Depression for diagnosis of depressive episodes.

E: MSE – hypomania and mania

A: Dress inappropriate/bright/outlandish. May be neglect of personal hygiene.

B: Overfamiliar, even flirtatious, increased psychomotor activity. Distractible, restless.

S: Loud, pressure of speech, uninterruptible, flight of ideas, puns and rhymes.

M: Euphoric but can quickly turn to irritability and anger.

T: *Abnormal thought tempo*: pressured thought.
Content: overvalued ideas.
Delusions: grandiose or persecutory.

P: Auditory hallucinations often mood congruent.

C: Attention and concentration often impaired.

I: Poor.

I: Exclude other causes for a manic episode: substance misuse, schizoaffective disorder, space-occupying lesion, hyperthyroidism, corticosteroids, anabolic androgenic steroids.

M:

Acute manic episode	Prophylaxis
• Most patients will require hospital admission – use of MHA if poor insight. • Lithium is a mood stabiliser. It takes 6–10 days to achieve full effects so antipsychotics are required for rapid control of acute behavioural disturbance. • A benzodiazepine may also be used as an adjunct. • Lithium may be started simultaneously. • ECT is less effective than antipsychotics. • Antidepressants can precipitate or aggravate a manic episode, so are stopped.	• Lithium and sodium valproate are mood stabilisers and are the main treatments used to prevent relapse. They help prevent both depression and mania; effective for 80% of sufferers. • Before lithium treatment is started check renal function, U&E, TFT and advise recontraception for women. Lithium has a narrow therapeutic range and therefore levels must be carefully monitored. See section on drug treatments. • It is important to educate the patient and family about lithium, its side-effects and signs of toxicity. Poor compliance can be a problem and the emphasis should be on patient support and clinical monitoring. • Carbamezapine and lamotrigine are also effective and may benefit some non-responders.

See Depression for management of depressive episodes.

C: 10% of those with BAD commit suicide.

Alcohol and substance misuse can complicate the picture; many with BAD self-medicate.

Non-compliance with lithium prophylaxis is an issue. Patients need to be on prophylaxis for life but often do not comply due to the side-effects or a prolonged period of well-being. Abrupt withdrawal of a mood stabiliser carries a high risk of relapse of mania and/or depression.

A minority of patients develop rapid cycling of four or more episodes a year. SRIs can trigger this.

P: The majority of those with BAD are well for most of the time as recovery between episodes is usually complete. Unfortunately, even with prolonged prophylaxis, 90% of patients will have at least one recurrence of mania and/or depression within 10 years.

The median duration of an untreated manic episode lasts 4 months. Depression lasts longer with a median duration of 6 months. With time, manic episodes tend to become less frequent and depressions are commoner and last longer.

Long-term prognosis can be poor as each relapse may be associated with hospitalisation, absence from work/education and strain on relationships. This accumulation of losses results in increased morbidity and mortality in those with BAD.

D: Eating disorder characterised by uncontrolled binge eating with vomiting/laxative abuse. Preoccupation with body weight and shape.

A: Dietary restraint triggers a cycle of binge followed by purging/starvation.

A/R: Depression, impulsivity, substance abuse. Many have previous history of AN.

E: Prevalence: 1–3%.
Sex ratio: F/M = 50 : 1.
Onset age: 15–30 years.

H: Binge eating up to 20 000 kcal in one session. They may feel a loss of control, or trance-like during binge. This is followed by self-loathing, vomiting and/or purging. Fasting, laxatives and diuretics are often abused.

E: Physical
signs of vomiting: pitted teeth, finger callus, parotid swelling
fluctuating (normal or excessive) weight
amenorrhoea in 50%

MSE
A&B: Anxious, defensive. May appear normal/excessive weight. Facial bloating due to parotid swelling.
S: Slow or normal.
M: Low, self-loathing.
T: Preoccupation with body weight and shape.
P: Usually no abnormal perceptions, although see themselves as fat even when not.
C: Concentration poor.
I: Variable.

I: U&E may show hypokalaemia and alkalosis due to vomiting.

M: (1) Medical stabilisation.
(2) Psychotherapy (CBT or CAT) to help re-establish a sensible eating pattern. Address underlying depression/low self-esteem.
(3) Drug therapies: SRI antidepressants have an antibulimic effect separate from their antidepressant effect, e.g fluoxetine.

C: Psychological
depression
re-feeding psychosis
OCD
deliberate self-harm
alcohol dependence
drug abuse
intense self-loathing

Laxative abuse: hypokalaemic alkalosis, cathartic colon.
Hypokalaemia: dysrhythmias, renal damage.
Acute oesophageal tears, oesophagogastritis, haematemesis.

P: Poor in patients with low BMI and with a high frequency of purging.
Short-term benefits of treatment well established.
CBT/CAT give remission in 50%.

ADULT PSYCHIATRIC DISORDERS

D: A term used to describe an idiopathic syndrome characterised principally by the occurrence of months of extreme disabling fatigue coupled with other somatic symptoms such as muscle pain and resulting in impairment of function. Other names that have been used in the past to describe these symptoms: ME, neurasthenia. ME was a term coined after an epidemic of unexplained symptoms and signs in the medical and nursing staff of the Royal Free Hospital in 1955. At first it was named 'Royal Free Disease'. The term ME continues to be used by some patients and doctors.

Fatigue has two components:
Physical
lack of energy
lack of interest in activities
muscular weakness

Mental
poor concentration and memory
lack of endurance
daytime sleepiness

Normal fatigue: occurring after mental or physical exercise with full recovery.
Abnormal fatigue: out of proportion to the level of exertion, slow to recover and which results in impairment of functioning.

A: Unknown and controversial, see below.

A/R: Anxiety and depression.
Chronic infection – patients often give a history of acute symptoms of viral infection. Symptoms often occur in epidemics (although these remain controversial – artificial linking by doctors and mass hysteria).
There is no evidence for an inflammation of the NS, as the term ME suggests.
Post-viral fatigue syndrome after EBV, but mostly this is considered as a separate condition.
Immune system dysfunction.
Candidiasis overgrowth in the gut.

E: It is thought that the prevalence of people complaining of fatigue at any one time is 20% of the population. However, only 1% can be considered as suffering from CFS.

H: Physical and mental fatigue must have been present for 6 months in order to make the diagnosis.

Core
feeling tired all the time
feeling tired easily
feeling excessively tired after activities
lack of energy

Biological
dizziness
inability to relax
irritability
aches and pains
decreased libido

Other symptoms often fluctuating
poor memory and concentration
depression

E: May be comorbid features of anxiety and depression.

All patients presenting with fatigue need a full physical examination.

I: Although the syndrome is idiopathic, investigations should be performed to exclude other pathology. It is best to keep an open mind.

FBC, ESR/CRP, U&E, glucose, TFT, anti-nuclear antibody tests should be routinely considered in all patients presenting with fatigue.

M: (1) Offer appropriate explanations, reassurance and hope, e.g. that the symptoms are genuinely disabling and not 'all in the mind', but that symptoms following exertion do not mean physical damage and long-term disability.

(2) For mild cases, patients can be advised to build up endurance gradually, starting with a manageable level and increasing a little each day.

(3) Give advice about sleeping patterns – encourage regular sleep pattern, avoid excessive rest/sudden changes in activity. Avoid drinking stimulants, e.g. caffeine, especially before bedtime.

(4) For more severe cases, patients may benefit from CBT based on a more formal exercise programme, and assessment using all the members of the MDT, e.g. physiotherapist, OT, psychologist.

(5) Antidepressant treatment will help for comorbid depression or anxiety.

C: Interrupts social functioning, e.g. relationship problems, unemployment. Suicide risk if comorbidity with depression.

P: Depends on severity. If mild symptoms, management in general practice may have a good outcome. Most are recovered by 2 years. However, if symptoms are severe and require hospital admission, the prognosis is poorer.

ADULT PSYCHIATRIC DISORDERS

D: Intentional self-inflicted injury/harm without a fatal outcome.
About 90% of cases involve drug overdose (e.g. paracetamol) and 10% involve self-injury (e.g. self-laceration of forearms/wrists).

A: Psychological

(1) Mixed and varied motives:
'cry for help'
to get relief
to escape a situation
to seek attention
to make someone feel guilty
(2) Impulsivity
(3) Poor coping strategies
(4) Self-punishment

A/F: Social

single/divorced
lower social classes
previous history of child abuse
unemployment
recent stressful event, e.g. loss of loved one, being in trouble with the law

Psychiatric

borderline personality disorder
depression (mild)
substance misuse
dysthymia

E: Incidence of 2–3/1000 in UK.
More prevalent in lower social classes.
Commoner in women.
Occurs in range of ages (teenagers to elderly) – commonest age group is the under 35.

I: Immediate risk of suicide.
Future/subsequent risk of suicide.
Clear picture of events that led to the episode (can be difficult as patients sometimes misrepresent intentions).
Current medical/psychosocial problems.
Coping strategies.

E: MSE – may reveal motives/features of psychiatric disorder.

E: None specifically.

M: (1) Treat as medically appropriate.
(2) Full assessment – assess risk and need for hospital admission. Use section 2 MHA if necessary.
(3) Interview should encourage patients to undertake a constructive review of their problems.
(4) Follow-up should be offered. Treatment of underlying psychiatric disorders.

Psychotherapy: psychodynamic, IPT, CBT (therapy involves resolving key problems that lead to the act and devising strategies to cope with future crises without resorting to self-harm, the emphasis is on self-help). Mood stabilisers, e.g. lithium, carbamazepine may reduce impulsivity.

C: Repeated self-harm, unintentional suicide, suicide.

P: 20% repeat the act within 1 year.
Risk of suicide within 1 year is 1–2%.
Poorer prognosis if severe family problems, history of previous self-harm.

ADULT PSYCHIATRIC DISORDERS

D: An acute, transient, global organic disorder of CNS function resulting in impaired consciousness and attention.

A: There are many causes for delirium.

Early	**Endocrine:** hypoglycaemia, DKA, thyroid dysfunction, Cushing's syndrome.
Management	**Metabolic:** hypoxia, electrolyte imbalance, dehydration, renal/liver/respiratory failure.
Is	**Infection:** systemic (UTI, pneumonia, HIV), local (encephalitis, meningitis, syphilis).
Very	**Vascular:** TIA/stroke.
Important	**Injury:** subdural haematoma, postconcussion.
For	**Food/nutrition:** thiamine deficiency.
Treating	**Tumours:** primary and secondary in the brain.
Delirium	**Drugs:** anaesthetic (post-operative), analgesics (opiates), anticholinergics, benzodiazepines, corticosteroids, digoxin, diuretics, EtOH.
Efficiently	**Epilepsy:** status epilepticus, post-ictal states.

A/R: Extremes of age (old and young), pre-existing dementia.

E 10% of all hospital inpatients; 30% of elderly hospital inpatients.

H: Often collateral history only. Previous mental state important.
Sudden onset, fluctuating consciousness.
Any symptoms of the underlying cause?
Hypo/hyperalert. Worse at night.
Hypersensitivity to light and sound.
Perceptual disturbance: misidentification, illusions and hallucinations
Reduced ability to maintain attention to external stimuli, and to shift attention to external stimuli appropriately.
Memory impairment, poor registration and retention of new material.

E MSE
A&B: Aggressive purposeless behaviour.
S: Incoherent, rambling.
M: Labile, anxious, depressed, irritable.
T: Disordered.
P: Illusions, hallucinations and distortions.
C: Poor, memory impairment, disoriented.
I: Poor.

Physical
Autonomic signs – sweating, tachycardia, dilated pupils.

I: Urine: screen for drugs, glucose and infection.
Blood: FBC, U&E, creatinine, glucose, LFT, TFT, CRP, blood cultures (if appropriate), ABG.
EEG: generalised slowing of background activity.
Depending on clinical findings, other investigations: CXR, SXR, HIV test, MRI/CT, LP.

M: Nursing management
Quiet and reassuring environment, good lighting.
Avoid frequent changes of staff.
Encourage relatives/friends to visit.

Medical

Reverse underlying cause if possible. Maintain adequate fluid and electrolyte balance.

Drugs: haloperidol for acute disturbances of behaviour, diazepam for alcohol withdrawal.

Consider use of the MHA if necessary.

Thiamine, nutrition.

P: Mortality can be high, up to 25% in elderly patients. Depends on the prognosis of the underlying cause, and rapidity of diagnosis and treatment.

It is important to distinguish between delirium and dementia, particularly in the elderly. However, dementia is a risk factor for delirium, and the two conditions can coexist. The table below highlights some of the differences.

Feature	Delirium	Dementia
Onset	Acute/subacute	Chronic/insidious
Course	Fluctuating	Stable, progressive
Attention	Markedly reduced	Normal, reduced
Arousal	Increased/decreased	Usually normal
Delusions	Fleeting	Systematised
Hallucinations	Common	Less common
Psychomotor activity	Usually abnormal	Usually normal
Autonomic features	Abnormal	Normal

ADULT PSYCHIATRIC DISORDERS

D: An organic syndrome characterised by gradual global deterioration of higher mental functioning without impairment of consciousness.

A: Commonest causes (accounting for more than 90% of all cases of dementia):

Alzheimer's disease
Vascular dementia
Diffuse Lewy body dementia
Pick's disease
Normal pressure hydrocephalus
Prion disease (CJD)

See organic psychiatry for other causes of reduced cognitive function.

A/R:

Type of dementia	Associated pathological findings	Genetic associations	Other
Alzheimer's disease	Generalised atrophy of the brain. Widening of the sulci and ventricles. Extracellular senile (beta-amyloid) plaques and intracellular neurofibrillary tangles. Reduced levels of neurotransmitters, e.g. ACh, NA, 5-HT.	E4 variant of apolipoprotein E gene. ? Autosomal dominant mutations causing early onset familial dementia. APP. Presenilin 1 & 2.	Age – increasing age is single most important risk factor. Family history. Down's syndrome associated with early onset dementia. Head injury.
Vascular dementia	Multiple white matter infarcts. Cystic necrosis of infarcted areas, reactive gliosis, patches of demyelisation of white matter.	Unknown.	Hypertension. Diabetes. Smoking. Male. Old age.
Lewy body dementia	Lewy bodies (eosinophilic intracellular structures) in cortical and subcortical neurones.	Unknown.	Parkinson's disease.

E: Prevalence of dementia: 1% in 65–74-year age group.
10% in > 75-year age group.
25% in > 85-year age group.

H: Often from a worried family member who has noticed changes in:
- **memory**, e.g. 'leaves the gas on and loses the door keys'
- **behaviour**, e.g. 'doesn't want to go out and visit friends anymore like always used to'
- **personality**, e.g. 'used to be a calm person, but now is very irritable and anxious'
- **mood change**, e.g. 'normally very cheerful but nothing seems to give pleasure anymore'

DIFFERENTIATING BETWEEN THE DEMENTIAS – THE MAIN FEATURES

Type of dementia	Age of onset & time course	Key clinical features
Alzheimer's disease	Onset usually after 65 years. Relentlessly progressive. Early onset, more rapid progression.	Short-term memory loss, difficulty learning/ retaining new information. Dysphasia, dyspraxia. Early impairment of sense of smell, persecutory beliefs are common.
Vascular dementia	Acute onset. Stepwise deterioration.	Memory loss, personality change, signs of vascular disease elsewhere.
Lewy body dementia	Average age of onset is 68 years. Variable rate of progression.	Fluctuating cognitive impairment. Visual hallucinations. Extrapyramidal symptoms (bradykinesia more than tremor). ? Sensitive to antipsychotics.
Frontotemporal dementia, e.g. Pick's disease	Insidious presenile onset usually between 50–60 years. Slow progression.	Early personality changes. Dementia with prominent frontal lobe involvement: coarsening of social behaviour, disinhibition, apathy/ restlessness. Memory is preserved in the early stages.
Normal pressure hydrocephalus	Average age of onset after 70 years.	Dementia with prominent frontal lobe dysfunction. Urinary incontinence. Gait disturbance.
CJD	Onset often before 65 years. Rapid progression – death within 2 years.	Affects all higher cerebral functions. Dementia associated with neurological signs: pyramidal, extrapyramidal, cerebellar, aphasia.

E: MSE will depend on the type of dementia. See the table above for distinguishing features.

I: Aimed at identifying aetiology.
Routine blood tests: FBC, U&E, B_{12} and folate, LFT.
More specialised blood tests: HIV, syphilis serology.
Radiology: CXR, brain imaging (CT or MRI).

ADULT PSYCHIATRIC DISORDERS

Neuropsychological testing (highlights brain regions affected/severity).
LP: CSF infection screen and pressure.
Specialised tests: genetic tests for familial dementia.
  brain biopsy and EEG for prion disease.
  cerebral blood flow tests.

M: (1) Explanation of nature of the illness and support for family, give information on support groups.
(2) Multi-disciplinary approach to diagnosis and assessment of specific needs.
(3) Deliver care – aim for maintaining dignity and individualisation.
Care package may include home help, day centres, respite residential stays.
Regular reassessment is needed to respond to changing needs.
(4) Physical treatments: cholinesterase inhibitors (donepezil) for mild cognitive and behavioural problems; may slow progression in Alzheimer's disease.
Severe behavioural problems may respond to low-dose antipsychotics.
Antidepressants for coexisting depression.

C: • Difficulty and distress for family – the main carer is often another elderly family member.
• Death often results due to pneumonia.
• There is a predisposition to delirium.

P: • The prognosis depends on the underlying cause.
• Younger age of onset usually means poorer prognosis.

Alzheimer's disease is usually fatal within 10 years of diagnosis.
Vascular dementia has a worse prognosis, with sudden stepwise deterioration and risk of sudden death from stroke.

D: Mood disorder characterised by a pervasive lowering of mood accompanied by psychosocial and biological symptoms. A typical depressive episode is described in terms of core symptoms, plus additional features (see history section below). A depressive episode may be further classified – depending on the severity of the symptoms and the impairment of social functioning – as mild, moderate, severe or severe with psychotic features. Symptoms present for at least 2 weeks.

A: Exact unknown.

Biological
genetic – 40% increased risk if family history
monoamine hypothesis – decrease in 5-HT, norepinephrine and DA
endocrine abnormalities, e.g. Cushing's syndrome, hypothyroidism

Psychosocial
stressful life events

A/R: **Vulnerable groups**
unemployed/low socio-economic status
divorced
single men
poor social support

Women
> 3 children under age 14
do not work outside the home
no one to confide in
separated from mother before age 11

Comorbidity with other psychiatric problems, e.g. alcohol misuse, anxiety disorders.

E:
- Common: point prevalence of depressive symptoms 15–20%.
- Lifetime risk: 10–20%. M/F = 1 : 2.
- Onset anytime from childhood to old age – median 30 years.

H: **Core**
low mood, typically worse AM
decreased enjoyment
fatigue and lethargy

Biological
psychomotor agitation/retardation
anhedonia
early morning wakening
loss of appetite and/or weight
loss of libido

Cognitive
Triad of pessimistic thoughts

(1) world – failure, see unhappy side of events
(2) future – expect worst, feel hopeless (suicidal)
(3) self – guilty, self-blame, reduced self-esteem

Additional
poor concentration and memory
poor sleep
tearfulness

If severe, patient may have mood-congruent psychotic symptoms, e.g. hallucinations and delusions. The main themes of these abnormal perceptions are worthlessness, guilt, ill health and poverty, e.g. patients may wrongly believe they have cancer, or that they have committed a crime and will be punished. Where delusions are persecutory, patients often believe that the punishment is deserved. Nihilistic delusions are an extreme form of depressive delusion.

Depressive stupor is an uncommon manifestation of depression characterised by a slowing of movement, and poverty of speech so extreme that the patient is motionless and mute.

E: MSE

A: Signs of neglect, e.g. weight loss, unkempt appearance.

B: Poor eye contact, downcast eyes, tearful.

S: Slow, non-spontaneous.

M: Low.

T: Pessimistic, suicidal, obsessions. Ideas/delusions of a hypochondriacal/ nihilistic nature.

P: Second-person auditory derogatory hallucinations.

C: Poor concentration.

I: Usually good.

Physical
May be signs of medical aetiology.

I: Blood tests to exclude medical cause, e.g. TFT, FBC, LFT, U&E, Ca, glucose.

M: (1) Risk assessment: suicide/neglect and explore psychosocial issues.
(2) Primary care if mild, psychiatric referral if severe, hospitalise if suicidal/psychotic.
(3) Drug treatments: antidepressants (TCA, SSRIs); lithium if refractory. ECT only if severe.
(4) Psychotherapies: supportive, CBT, IPT.

C: Social isolation, unemployment, self-harm/suicide, drug/alcohol abuse, chronic dysthymia.

P: For major depressive episode: average 6-month duration, lifetime suicide risk 15%, recurrence rate up to 80%.

OTHER DEPRESSIVE SYNDROMES

Atypical depression – a term that has been applied to a variety of presentations, but particularly to patients who present with mild to moderate depression, some mood reactivity, reverse diurnal variation in mood (i.e. worse in the evening), overeating, hypersomnia and fatigue.

Dysthymia – depressive symptoms which are insufficient to meet the criteria for a clinical depression. The patient's symptoms are present for 2 or more years. Can be associated with other psychiatric conditions such as borderline personality disorder. Sufferers often go on to develop more serious mood disorder.

Cyclothymic disorder – chronic mood fluctuations over at least 2 years with episodes of elation and of depression insufficient to meet the criteria for a hypomanic depressive episode.

Masked depression – a state in which depressed mood is not particularly prominent, but other features of depressive disorder are present, e.g. sleep disturbance, diurnal mood variation, depressive cognitions.

Mild depressive disorders – milder forms of the symptoms of depression, with less disruption to social functioning. These are likely to be accompanied by prominent anxiety, phobic or obsessional symptoms.

Recurrent brief depressive disorder – lasts for <2 weeks, usually around 2–3 days. Occurs around once per month, with complete recovery between episodes. The actual symptoms collectively may fulfil the criteria for mild, moderate or severe depression, but the difference is in the duration of the episode.

SAD – a temporal relationship between the season of the year and the onset of depression. The depression starts in autumn/winter and resolves in spring/summer. There may be symptoms of depression and additional atypical biological features such as carbohydrate craving, fatigue and hypersomnia.

ADULT PSYCHIATRIC DISORDERS

ADULT PSYCHIATRIC DISORDERS

D: A general definition is physical symptoms (or mental symptoms) that occur without the physical pathology usually associated with them. However, DSM-IV and ICD-10 differ in their classification of the symptoms. In DSM-IV, dissociative disorders refer to mental symptoms and conversion disorders refer to physical symptoms. ICD-10 refers to both types of symptoms as dissociative disorders, and the terms dissociative and conversion disorder may be used interchangeably. We have followed the ICD practice in the lists below.

A: Used to be called hysteria – the ancient Greeks thought it was due to the movement of the uterus (hysterus) into an abnormal position! Now thought to be due to an innate biological mechanism that counteracts highly stressful experiences. Becomes chronic either because deliberately cultivated or habit.

A/R: There are convincing associations in time with stressful life events, problems or needs. Depression also has an association.

E: Rare disorder. 3–6/1000 women. Less common in men. Most cases begin before age 35 years.

H: The symptoms usually confer some advantage on the patient, e.g. reduced workload/responsibility. Called 'secondary gain'. The patients often show less distress than would be expected of someone with their symptoms, sometimes called 'belle indifférence'. However, they often show exaggerated emotional reactions to other things.

Must be distinguished from malingering, in which the patient consciously and deliberately feigns illness in order to avoid a situation, e.g. prison.

Types of dissociative state:

- Dissociative amnesia – unable to recall long periods of their life.
- Dissociative fugue – lose their memory and wander away from their usual surroundings, deny any memory of where they went.
- Dissociative pseudodementia – the patient shows abnormality of intelligence suggesting dementia, but answers questions wrongly in a way that suggests they have the correct answer in mind, e.g. the Ganser question: 'how many legs does a cow have?' answer, '3' or '5'!
- Dissociative stupor – motionless and mute, but they are aware of their surroundings.
- Dissociative identity disorder (also known as multiple personality disorder) – sudden alternations between two patterns of behaviour, each of which is forgotten by the patient when the other is present.
- Dissociative anaesthesia or sensory loss – often with unusual distribution of loss of sensation, e.g. hands only (includes hysterical blindness).
- Dissociative convulsions (also known as pseudoseizures) – serum prolactin *not* elevated when sample taken 20 minutes after a 'fit', whereas in genuine seizures prolactin is raised.

E: There must be *no evidence* of a physical disease that can explain the symptoms of this disorder.

MSE

A&B: Depends on the type of dissociation. Loss of function.

S: Normal, unless they are mute (as in dissociative stupor).

M: May be low, depressed.

T: Surprisingly unconcerned about their disability.

C: May be impaired.

I: Poor.

I: Exclude physical cause for the symptoms. This may be difficult.

M: Accept that the patients' symptoms are real to them. Encourage them to get better.

If there are still stressful problems/life events, aim to deal with these factors. Physical rehabilitation may help. Treat depression.

C: These conditions may become chronic because of deliberate cultivation for the secondary gain, or simply become habit.

P: Variable.

ADULT PSYCHIATRIC DISORDERS

D: Discrete, recurrent abnormality in electrical activity of the brain resulting in behavioural, motor or sensory changes, or changes in consciousness.

A: Unknown.

A/R: Family history.

E: Prevalence of active epilepsy is 1%.

H: Prodrome: irritability, tension, restlessness, insomnia, occasional suicidal depression. May occur days or hours before fit.

Ictal: aura – only for localised fits. May experience acute perceptual changes, depersonalisation, acute mood changes, rising epigastric feelings.

Post-ictal: confusional state. May even experience transient paranoid hallucinations.

E: May have clouded consciousness, simple or complex movements or actions.

I: Exclude other causes for fits, e.g. post-traumatic, cerebrovascular, space-occupying lesions, drug/alcohol withdrawal, hypoglycaemia, hypoxia, encephalitis, syphilis, HIV.

Diagnosis on clinical grounds. EEG between episodes may be normal, but may help localise the focus.

M: Medication depends on type of epilepsy. Examples of anti-epileptic drugs are sodium valproate and carbamazepine.

Treat depression. Advise the patient not to drive until fits are under control, i.e. 1 year seizure-free.

C: Between fits may show aggressive behaviour; depression and suicide are more common in non-dominant temporal lobe lesions.

Schizophreniform psychosis is associated with temporal lobe epilepsy.

P: Mortality risk higher in epileptics than healthy controls.

D: Persistent and generalised anxiety about everyday events, not restricted to a particular situation or phobic stimulus. Present for at least 6 months for diagnosis.

A: **Biological**
genetic predisposition
autonomic nervous system abnormalities (increased sympathetic tone)

Psychosocial
current stress
life events

A/R: Childhood experiences characterised by separations, demands for high achievement and excess conformity.

E: Lifetime prevalence 5%. F > M.

Onset adolescence to early adulthood.

H: Fears which are excessive, disproportionate and unfocused.
Increased vigilance, restless, on edge.
Insomnia/middle insomnia/fatigue on waking.
Motor tension – tremors, headache.
Autonomic hyperactivity (arousal, sweating, increased HR, RR, dilated pupils).
Prolonged course, relapses and remissions, may or may not be a reaction to external events.

I: Increased HR, increased skin conductance, increased forearm blood flow and muscular tension. Hyperactive deep reflexes.

EEG may show reduced alpha rhythm.

M: (1) Reassurance, counselling and psychotherapy.
(2) CBT to identify anticipatory anxieties and replace them with realistic cognitions.
(3) Anxiety management training, e.g. relaxation therapy.
(4) Treat comorbid conditions, e.g. depression, somatoform disorders.
(5) Drug therapies: short-term benzodiazepines, TCAs, beta blockers.

C: Secondary agoraphobia, depression, alcohol/drug abuse.

P: Course may be chronic, worse at times of stress.

ADULT PSYCHIATRIC DISORDERS

D: Choreiform involuntary movements.

A: Autosomal dominant. Chromosome 4. Too few GABA–ergic and cholinergic neurones in the corpus striatum.

A/R: Family history (or may very occasionally be a new mutation).

E: 4–7/100 000. M = F. Usual onset age 25–50 years.

H: Psychiatric symptoms common: depression, behaviour change/irritability schizophreniform psychosis, dementia.
The chorea is followed eventually by dementia, seizures and death.

E: MSE
A&B: Abnormal movements.
S: Normal.
M: May be low.
T: Normal.
P: None.
C: Impaired in dementia.
I: Insight may be good preceding dementia.

E: Genetic tests.

M: Symptomatic treatment. Children of an affected parent have a 50% chance of inheriting the condition. Relatives may wish to be tested and require genetic counselling.

C: Suicide risk for patient and their relatives.

P: A neurodegenerative condition. No treatment can prevent progression.

D: Male hypogonadism due to having 47 chromosomes (XXY) or 48 (XXYY).

A: Polysomy and variable Leydig cell defect.

A/R: Reduced thyroxine levels, diabetes, asthma.

E: 1/600 live births.

I: Mild intellectual impairment, personality/behaviour problems, sexual problems, psychosis.

S: Small testes, penis, gynaecomastia, female pubic hair pattern, oligospermia, infertility, androgen deficiency.

I: Chromosomal testing.

M: Androgens, surgery for gynaecomastia.

C: Alcohol dependency, criminal behaviour.

P: Normal life expectancy.

ADULT PSYCHIATRIC DISORDERS

ADULT PSYCHIATRIC DISORDERS

D: Lower and upper motor neurone degeneration. No sensory symptoms and it never affects external ocular movements.

A: Unknown.

A/R: ? Viruses, e.g. polio.

E: Onset age 50–60 years. Affects 7/10 000. M/F $= 3 : 2$.

H: Stumbling, spastic gait, foot-drop. Upper and lower motor neurone signs on examination. No sensory symptoms.
Sleep disturbance, fatigue.

E: MSE
A&B: May be fatigued, depressed.
S: Normal, depending on cranial nerves being intact.
M: Emotional lability.
T: Normal.
P: Normal.
C: Mild cognitive deficits may progress to dementia.
I: Good.

I: MRI, LP to exclude structural/inflammatory causes.

M: Treat symptoms, e.g. baclofen for spasticity. Treat depression. Pain control with narcotics may be needed.

C: Frontal lobe dementia.

P: Progressive disease. Most die within 5 years of diagnosis.

D: Relapsing and remitting chronic disease due to plaques of demyelination and axon loss throughout the CNS.

A: Unknown.

A/R: Temperate areas.

E: F > M. 20–40 years peak age of onset. 40/100 000 prevalence.

H: Physical
fatigue
motor weakness/spasticity
numbness
urinary frequency
urgency
incontinence
constipation
sexual dysfunction
swallowing disorders
visual disturbances
vertigo

Psychiatric
transient mood changes
irritability
anxiety
intellectual impairments
depression (may be reactive)
euphoria (elevation of mood out of keeping with the patient's physical disability)
emotional lability

Psychosis, hysteria and hypomania are rare.

E: MSE
A&B: May be anxious, irritable.
S: Normal.
M: Low or may be euphoric.
T: Usually normal.
P: None.
C: Impaired memory, attention, abstract thinking.
I: Good.

I: MRI scan may show plaques of demyelination.
CSF shows increased protein and oligoclonal IgG bands on electrophoresis.

M: Methylprednisolone, baclofen (for muscle spasms), beta interferon.
Treat psychiatric symptoms appropriately.

C: Psychosis (rare).

P: Progressive disease. Prognosis worse if older, male or have many early relapses/early disability.

D: An anxiety disorder in which the patients suffer from egodystonic time-consuming obsessions and compulsions, which interfere with normal everyday life. The patients recognise that their thoughts are excessive and usually try to resist them, unsuccessfully.

A: *Psychoanalytic theory*: obsessions are used to prevent undesirable ideas entering consciousness, e.g. unconscious conflicts (sexual and aggressive).
Behavioural theory: compulsions decrease anxiety, so the condition is reinforced.
Biological theory:
• genetic influence – positive family history in 50%.
• 5-HT abnormalities.
• Frontal cortex and basal ganglia abnormalities.

A/R: Single. Anankastic premorbid personality traits found in 70%. Comorbid depression is present in 30% of OCD patients. Symptoms are also exacerbated by depression. Many life events in the year prior to onset.

E: Lifetime prevalence 2–3%. M = F. Age of onset usually by early twenties.

H: Obsessions and compulsions present on most days for a period of 2 weeks. They cause distress and interfere with the patient's life.
Obsessions may be persistent thoughts, images, doubts or impulses. Content may be repugnant, worrying, blasphemous, obscene:
• dirt/contamination
• sex
• aggression
• religion
• socially unacceptable actions
• orderliness
Compulsions are stereotyped acts, recognised as excessive, unreasonable or exaggerated. If the patient tries to resist doing them, there is a sense of mounting tension that can be immediately relieved by yielding to the compulsion. Often involve cleaning, repeating, checking, orderliness, hoarding. Compulsions may also take the form of mental rituals to decrease anxiety, e.g. counting in 4s.

E: Poor concentration if distracted by unwanted thoughts. May show signs of increasing anxiety if prevented from yielding to compulsions.
They recognise that the thoughts are their own and excessive.

I: None specifically.

M: (1) Treat comorbid medical and psychiatric conditions (e.g. depression).
(2) Exposure and response prevention – CBT.
(3) Habituation training and thought stopping for obsessions.
(4) Drug therapy: SRIs, clomipramine, antipsychotics may be useful in treatment-resistant OCD.
(5) Psychosurgery rarely used, for refractory cases.

C: Difficulty with relationships, work and social functioning. Waxing and waning course. Increased risk of suicide.

P: 2/3 respond to treatment. Worse prognosis if severe symptoms, premorbid obsessional personality disorder, life stresses.

D: Reduced dopaminergic activity in the striatum causing movement disorders: tremor, rigidity, bradykinesia and difficulty starting and stopping walking.

A: Degeneration of dopaminergic neurones in the substantia nigra.

A/R: Mitochondrial mutations resulting in reduced ATP. Pesticides and toxins have also been implicated as possible causes. (Neuroleptics and Wilson's disease may cause a similar Parkinsonian syndrome.)

E: Affects 0.5% of the population over 65 years.
Age of onset: usually 50–70 years.

H: Resting tremor, rigidity, slow movement, monotonous speech, shuffling steps (festinant gait).

Psychiatric symptoms are common, including:
depressive symptoms (reactive or due to neurotransmitter abnormalities) in 70%
cognitive deficits in 10–20%
psychoses (due to long-term treatment)

E: MSE
A&B: Masklike face, reduced facial expressions.
S: Slow, monotonous.
M: Depression in many.
T: Rarely have psychotic symptoms, e.g. paranoid delusions.
P: Rarely may have abnormal perceptions.
C: 10–20% have cognitive deficits.
I: Variable.

E: Clinical diagnosis. Exclude medication as the cause of Parkinsonism.

M: Atypical antipsychotics for psychosis – these are less likely to induce extrapyramidal side-effects.
Treat depression – nortriptyline is least likely to worsen Parkinson's disease.
DA agonists for the movement disorder – L-dopa.

C: Depression, suicide, dementia.

P: Progressive condition.

ADULT PSYCHIATRIC DISORDERS

D: Disorders characterised by an enduring, deeply ingrained pervasive and inflexible pattern of inner experience and behaviour, which are maladaptive in the individual's culture and lead to distress or impairment of work or social functioning.

A: Exact unknown – may vary between types.

Biological
genetics (e.g. *D4DR* gene related to novelty-seeking behaviour)
abnormal brain maturation during early years in life
underactive autonomic nervous system

A/R: **General**
social reinforcement of abnormal behaviours
low social class
poor parenting
disrupted/arrested psychic development

Borderline personality disorder – dysfunctional families, sexual abuse.

E: 3–5% of adult population have a PD.
Age of onset: adolescence/early adulthood.

H: Maladaptions may manifest as

- cognitions
- affectivity
- control over impulses and gratification of needs
- manner of relating to others
- handling of interpersonal situations
- manner of handling stress

PDs are divided into 3 clusters.
A = Odd/Eccentric
Paranoid – sensitivity, suspicious, self-reference, bears grudges, jealous.
Schizoid – cold, aloof, introspective, lacks social norms, withdrawn and detached, little interest in sexual experience.
B = Dramatic/Emotional
Histrionic – egocentric, shallow mood, self-dramatisation – likes to be centre of attention.
Dissocial – No tolerance. Blames others. No guilt, callous unconcern for others, irritability, tendency to violence (also known as psychopathic disorder, psychopathy, sociopathy).
Emotionally unstable: (1) impulsive – inability to plan ahead, unstable mood etc. (2) borderline – empty, unclear self-image, repeated self-harm, parasuicide. Chronic feelings of emptiness, fear of abandonment.
C = Fearful/Anxious
Anankastic – obsessional, pedantic, perfectionist, cautious, needs to plan ahead with meticulous detail.
Dependent – needs reassurance, will not take responsibility, feels inadequacy, fear of abandonment.
Anxious – feeling of tension and apprehension, fear of criticism or rejection, self-conscious.

E: MSE will vary depending on the features above.

I: Personality Diagnostic Questionnaire (PDQ), Structured Clinical Interview for PD (SCIPD), Standardised Assessment of Personality (SAP), International Personality Disorder Examination (IPDE).
MRI to exclude organic causes of personality change, e.g. frontal lobe tumour, subdural haematoma.

M: (1) Careful assessment should be conducted – need collateral history.
(2) Treatment of comorbid psychiatric disorders, e.g. depression.
(3) Psychotherapies: dynamic/CBT; individual/group therapy.
(4) Drug therapies: low-dose antipsychotics for ideas of reference, impulsivity and intensely angry affect.
Antidepressants may be useful in borderline personality disorder.
Carbamazepine + lithium may be used for episodic behavioural dyscontrol and aggression.
(5) May require detention under MHA if dangerous and violent or suicide risk.
(6) Therapeutic communities, e.g. Henderson Hospital.

C: Subjective distress. Adverse effects on relationships/society. Alcohol and substance abuse. Increased suicide risk.

P: There is evidence that cluster B mature with time. Likely to impair social or work functioning.

Personality type	Prognosis
Paranoid	Poor, many continue to have marital, social and occupational difficulties.
Schizoid	Poor, relationship to schizophrenia is uncertain.
Dissocial	Variable prognosis, may improve with age. Comorbid problems, e.g. abuse of drugs/EtOH, forensic history result in worse outcome.
Histrionic	May improve with age. Abuse of alcohol and drugs has a poorer prognosis.
Borderline	May improve with age. Abuse of substances is associated with a poorer outcome. Increased suicide risk.
Anxious	May develop social phobia. Protected environment has a favourable outcome.
Dependent	Good outcome with treatment. Loss of the person they are dependent on has a poorer prognosis.
Anankastic	May go on to develop OCD, may do well at jobs requiring obsessional behaviour, no improvement with age.

ADULT PSYCHIATRIC DISORDERS

D: Also known as maternity blues, baby blues. A common psychological problem occurring typically around the 3rd day post partum consisting of emotional and behavioural disturbances.

It is not a psychiatric disorder and should not be considered abnormal; however, it is included because it is common and must be distinguished from postnatal depression, which is a psychiatric disorder.

A: Unknown.

Biological theories suggest hormonal changes after birth: decrease in oestrogen and progesterone; fluid and electrolyte changes.

A/R:
- Increased incidence in women who have previously suffered severe PMS.
- Commoner in primigravidae.

E: Occurs in over 50% of mothers.

H: Symptoms begin within the first 10 days post partum, typically from the 3rd to 5th day, and resolve spontaneously within a few days.

Psychological
emotional lability
low mood
anxious (fear of inability to cope)

Behavioural
irritability
crying
decreased sleep

E: MSE – features may be similar to mild depression and anxiety.

I: Not appropriate.

M: (1) Reassurance, explanation and family support are the key features.
(2) Antenatal education that gives warning for women and their partner is helpful.

C: May upset early bonding and breastfeeding.

P: Good, self-limiting within a few days.

D: Also known as puerperal depression. Depression arising within a year of childbirth.
NB: Postnatal depression is a different entity from the normal baby blues.

A:
- Exact unknown.
- Psychosocial factors play a major role, e.g. lack of support. The depression usually starts after the woman has left hospital and has been discharged by the midwife.
- Biological theories suggest hormonal changes: sudden drop in oestrogen and progesterone levels.

A/R:
- Recent stressful life event.
- Past psychiatric history, especially depression.
- Emotional instability immediately after birth.
- Family history of postnatal depression.
- Residual pain.

E: Affects 10% of mothers.

H:
- Usually occurs within 2–6 weeks of delivery.
- May have developed insidiously over several weeks or as an exacerbation of the baby blues.
- Similar features to general depressive illness.

- In addition, note:
  Sleep disturbance, energy changes and low libido are less sensitive indicators as these can occur normally after a birth.
  Cognitive features are more sensitive indicators and are usually based around motherhood, e.g. feels guilty for not coping as a mother; gains no pleasure from the child; feels angry with child.
  Tearfulness, poor concentration and feeling anxious are common symptoms.

E: MSE – see Depression.
T: Overvalued ideas (e.g. thinks she is unable to look after the child).
Obsessional thoughts (e.g. fears harm will come to child).
Pessimistic.
Suicidal.
Infanticidal.

I: As for depression.

M:
(1) Assess risk to mother and child.
(2) Most cases can be managed at home, although if severe admit to mother and baby unit (may need to use MHA).
(3) Multi-disciplinary care – liaise with GP and midwife/health visitor.
(4) Give reassurance and provide supportive measures, counselling/CBT.
(5) Give information about support groups, e.g. local mothers' group.
(6) Antidepressant medication – see prescribing in breastfeeding.
(7) Screening for depression should be incorporated into 6-week postnatal check.

C:
- Bonding failure.
- Rejection/neglect of the baby.
- Marital/relationship problems.
- Child development and behavioural problems later on.
- Maternal suicide or infanticide.

P: 90% of cases last less than 1 month with treatment, 4% are still depressed 1 year later.

ADULT PSYCHIATRIC DISORDERS

D: Intense, prolonged, delayed reaction to an exceptionally stressful event.

A: Traumatic events, e.g. being victim of violence or personal attack, observer/survivor of civilian disasters, being involved in combat.
The event must have been significant enough to cause distress in almost anyone.
Cognitive theories – key points:

- The event challenges currently held beliefs, this results in an inability to cognitively rationalise the event.
- Normal processing of emotionally charged information is overwhelmed so memories persist in an unprocessed form, which can intrude into conscious awareness.
- Negative appraisal of intrusive thoughts maintains experience of symptoms over time.

A/R: Biological
genetic vulnerability
borderline/dependent personality disorder
being female

Psychosocial
acquired vulnerability
previous traumatic event (especially as a child)
recent experience of stressful life events

E: Lifetime risk up to 14% for general population and 58% for at-risk groups. High prevalence in asylum seekers and refugees.

H: Occurs weeks/months after the event, onset usually within 6 months.
Symptoms must have been present for 1 month in order to make the diagnosis.
3 main groups of symptoms (not present before the exposure)

(1) **Hyperarousal**
persistent anxiety
hypervigilence
poor concentration
insomnia
(2) **Intrusions**
flashbacks
distressing dreams
vivid memories
(3) **Avoidance**
avoids reminders
inability to recall some of the events
poor interest in everyday life

May be comorbid depressive symptoms, alcohol and drug abuse.

E: MSE – overlap with depression and anxiety.
A: May be signs of neglect related to depression, may look anxious, hypervigilance.
B: Poor eye contact, tearful.
S: Slow, non-spontaneous.
M: Low, anxious.
T: Pessimistic, suicidal.
P: Illusions related to anxiety.

C: Concentration may be poor.

I: Usually good.

I: None specifically.

M: (1) Screen for comorbid psychiatric disorders and conduct risk assessment (suicide/neglect).

(2) Referral to support groups, e.g. Medical Foundation for Victims of Torture.

(3) Psychotherapies – crisis counselling, CBT, debriefing (recall of the event with emotional support), eye movement desensitising and re-processing.

(4) Drug treatments – antidepressants, short-term benzodiazpines.

C: Social withdrawal, suicide.

P: Depends on duration and severity of the symptoms. About half make good recovery within 1 year of onset, others may have lifelong symptoms.

ADULT PSYCHIATRIC DISORDERS

Premenstrual syndrome

ADULT PSYCHIATRIC DISORDERS

D: Also known as PMS. A syndrome comprising psychological, behavioural and physical symptoms that are cyclical, starting in the luteal phase (days 14–28) of the menstrual cycle and ending during menstruation (days 1–4).
It is not considered a psychiatric disorder; however, it is included because it is a common problem that presents in general practice and if severe may require treatment with SRI antidepressants.

A: Unknown.
Biological theories have been suggested. Changes in ovarian function and hormone levels may result in neurotransmitter imbalances or fluid and electrolyte imbalances.

A/R: None specifically, apart from being a woman!
PMS may be a presenting feature of depression.

E: Up to 90% of women experience cyclical symptoms.
Only 3% experience disabling symptoms.
Onset after menarche.

H: Symptoms must have cyclical nature.
Biological
bloated feeling
acne
headache
stomach cramps
breast tenderness
weight gain

Psychological
anxiety
tiredness
depression

Behavioural
irritability
aggression
loss of control

Always enquire about suicidal feelings.

E: • Depends on point in menstrual cycle.
• PMS may give a picture similar to mild depression/anxiety.

I: Clinical diary of menstrual symptoms.

M: (1) No treatments have proved to be effective in all women and some tried are thought to have a high placebo effect.
(2) If symptoms are mild, CBT and relaxation therapy may be helpful to provide mechanisms for coping during this part of the cycle.
(3) Pharmacotherapies: evening primrose oil, vitamin B_6 and the combined oral contraceptive pill have been found to be helpful.
(4) For severe symptoms, if the above are unhelpful, antidepressants of the SRI class have been found to be helpful.

C: Interference with daily living, e.g. time off work.

P: Persistent problem for a small percentage of women.

D: ICD-10 categories of psychosexual disorder
- Sexual dysfunction, e.g. erectile/ejaculatory failure, dyspareunia, vaginismus, orgasmic dysfunction.
- Sexual preference, e.g. paraphilias: paedophilia, fetishism, transsexism, bestiality, necrophilia, exhibitionism, sadomasochism.
- Gender identity disorder.
- Sexual problems as part of a psychiatric disorder, e.g. depression.

A: Sexual dysfunction
Connections between physical state and feelings about sexuality/function. Cannot separate the physical from the psychological.
Physical
Hormonal – low testosterone, low oestrogen (menopause).
Local – prostate surgery (often causes retrograde ejaculation), bladder surgery, colostomy, gynaecological surgery, mastectomy (psychological effects of surgery), STDs.
Systemic – diabetes, hypertension, neurological disease, e.g. multiple sclerosis.
Drugs – medical. Beta blockers (delay erection), ACE inhibitors, diuretics, phenytoin, antidepressants, metoclopramide and the older antipsychotics (both increase prolactin which causes decreased sexual drive), cimetidine, HRT.
Drugs – recreational. Alcohol (disinhibiting in small amounts, can lead to decreased arousal and erectile failure; long-term use causes ovarian and testicular atrophy and neuropathy).

Psychological
Negative emotions and fears related to past experiences, e.g. child sexual abuse/rape.
Recent life events, e.g. bereavement, diagnosis of cancer, divorce, unemployment, new sexual partner, childbirth, termination of pregnancy, miscarriage, infertility, diagnosis of STD.
Parental/cultural influences and conditioning.
Religious influences, e.g. associate sex with guilt.
Difficulties within relationship with sexual partner.
Psychiatric disorders, e.g. depression, anxiety.

A/R: Men tend to present with erectile/ejaculatory dysfunction while women commonly present with dyspareunia/vaginismus/decreased sexual drive/orgasmic dysfunction.

E: Up to 20% of women and 30% of men complain of sexual dysfunction.
20% of men over the age of 65 report erectile dysfunction.
Incidence of gender identity disorders: < 3/100 000 males and < 1/100 000 females.

H: Full history – symptoms, functional problem (situational links?), gynaecological history in women, sexual history, previous medical history including STDs. Organic primary problem or secondary psychological problem (can coexist).
Beware of assuming gender preference – use term 'your partner' if uncertain.

E: MSE – look for features of depression, guilt, anxiety.

I: Exclude organic cause for sexual dysfunction, e.g. STDs.

ADULT PSYCHIATRIC DISORDERS

M: **Psychological**
Brief psychosexual therapy.
CBT – challenging assumptions, sexual re-education, communication training, setting goals, anxiety reduction.
Masters & Johnson–based behavioural therapy – couples are given hierarchy of sexual 'assignments' (homework), keeping within agreed limits, aiming to identify problems, e.g. feelings, anxiety, attitudes.
Couples therapy for relationship problems.
Psychotherapy for long-standing, deep-seated problems.

Medical
For erectile dysfunction:
sildefanil
alprostadil (intracavernosal self-injections)
yohimbine (alpha-2 antagonist)
testosterone supplements if levels low
oestrogen HRT
vacuum pumps
surgical implants

C: Many transsexuals have coexisting psychological pathology and are prone to depression/suicide. This can be marked post-operatively when gender reassignment surgery may not fulfil all expectations. Pre- and post-surgical psychological assessment and counselling is therefore vital.

P: Variable. Good prognostic factors include stable relationship, high motivation and early referral for treatment.

D: A psychotic disorder arising within 1 year of childbirth.

A: Exact unknown.
Biological theories implicate
- genetic factors (risk is increased if there is family history)
- hormonal factors (sudden drop in oestrogen following delivery)
- supersensitivity of DA receptors

A/R: Past history of psychosis/mood disorder.
Primigravida.

E: Affects 0.1% of mothers.

H:
- Usually arises within 4 weeks of delivery.
- Features may be of depression, schizophrenia or more commonly mania – see relevant chapters.
- Special features include:
  acute onset of symptoms
  may be a prodrome of insomnia and psychomotor agitation
  fluctuating symptoms, e.g. labile mood
  rational periods giving deception of recovery
  poor memory and confusion

E: MSE – see Depression, Schizophrenia, Mania.
Perceptions and abnormal thoughts are mainly based around the infant.
T: Paranoid delusions, e.g. is convinced that her baby has been swapped with someone else's.
P: Persecutory auditory hallucinations, e.g. hears voice of the baby as voice of the devil.
Command auditory hallucinations, e.g. voices instructing her to kill the baby.
Physical examination – to rule out delirium due to infection.

I: To rule out infection.

M: (1) Risk assessment of mother and child.
(2) Admit to hospital (preferably mother and baby unit) if appropriate (using section 2 MHA), rarely manage at home with frequent review involving health visitors and CPN.
(3) Physical treatments include drug therapy for the appropriate clinical situation (antidepressants, antipsychotics, lithium) and ECT, which may be effective for pharmacologically refractory cases.
(4) Counselling/psychotherapy may be helpful during recovery to help the woman come to terms with and understand the nature of the illness, and to allow her to eliminate any feelings of guilt or failure.

C:
- Harm/neglect of the child.
- Suicide/infanticide.

P: Most recover and the short-term prognosis is good. However, the recurrence rate is 50% for subsequent non-puerperal psychosis and 25% for subsequent puerperal psychosis.

ADULT PSYCHIATRIC DISORDERS

D: A chronic psychotic disorder.

ICD-10: diagnosis requires the presence of at least two of: delusions, hallucinations, disorganised speech, disorganised thought, disorganised behaviour for 1 month or at least 1 year of negative symptoms. In the absence of organic disease, alcohol or drug-related dependence/ withdrawal. Not secondary to elevation or depression of mood.

ICD-10 subgroups of schizophrenia: paranoid (persecutory or grandiose features); hebephrenic (irresponsible/unpredictable); catatonic (catatonic symptoms); simple (insidious decline in function); residual (chronic negative symptoms).

A: Multifactorial. Currently believed to be a genetically driven neurodevelopmental disorder.

Genetic: Monozygotic twins have a 48% chance of concordance. Increased risk in people who have a first-degree relative with schizophrenia.

Environment: Obstetric birth complications or *in utero* exposure to viral agent(s) leading to aberrant early brain development.

Neurochemical: Older theories focused on defects in the DA system, newer theories include hypofunction in glutaminergic neurotransmission involving hippocampal NMDA receptors.

Brain structural changes: Imaging studies show decreased cortical volume, especially of the temporal lobe, and enlargement of the lateral ventricles.

A/R: **Precipitants**
Stress, psychoactive drugs.

Vulnerable groups
Single, family history of schizophrenia.

Poor prognosis
Abnormal premorbid personality, low IQ, early age at onset, insidious onset, absence of any obvious precipitant, absence of positive symptoms, high EE in family.

Good prognosis
Presence of mood component.

E: Point prevalence: 0.25–0.5%. M/F = 1 : 1.
Lifetime risk: 0.7–0.9%.
Median age of onset: males 28 years, females 32 years.

H: Schizophrenia is a chronic disease and involves more than one psychotic episode. The more clinical features there are, the more likely a diagnosis of schizophrenia becomes. Often has a prodromal period of decline in performance (e.g. at school, university, work) with social withdrawal.

E: MSE

Positive signs & symptoms	Negative signs & symptoms
A: Normal or inappropriate dress, headgear, etc.	A: Poor self-care/unkempt.
B: Withdrawn or restless and noisy.	B: Tardive dyskinesia/poor eye contact/apathy.
M: Flattened/inappropriate/anxious/ guarded/depressed.	M: Flattened/blunted.
S: Reflects underlying thought disorder.	S: Poverty of speech.
T: *Formal thought disorder*: derailment, loosening of associations, thought blocking. *Thought alienation*: broadcasting, withdrawal, insertion. *Delusions*: persecutory/reference/ control/grandiose.	T: May be formal thought disorder, may be persistent delusions.
P: Third-person auditory hallucinations, especially in the form of a running commentary, hallucinations in other senses.	P: May have persistent auditory hallucinations.
C: Orientation often normal, impaired attention & concentration.	C: Specific cognitive deficits.
I: Poor.	I: Poor.

Groupings of symptoms that have been previously used:

Schneiderian first-rank symptoms
(1) Delusional perception: abnormal belief attached to a normal perception, arising *de novo*.
(2) Third-person auditory hallucinations: thought echo, running commentary.
(3) Thought interference: thought withdrawal, insertion, broadcast.
(4) Passivity phenomenon: individuals believe that their actions are being controlled externally.

Bleuler's 4 As
Autistic thoughts – inner world of fantasy.
Affective incongruity – e.g. smiling when describing a sad event.
Associations loosened – thought disorder.
Ambivalence – conflicting feelings.

I: Exclude organic cause.
Blood: FBC, TFT, glucose, U&E, B_{12} and folate, VDRL.
Drug levels: substance misuse?
If neurological symptoms/signs or if first episode: brain imaging and EEG.
Neuropsychological testing for first episode.

M: Involve family/carers, as they need to be supported and educated about the illness.
(1) Risk assessment: suicidality/need for hospitalisation/detention under MHA? CPA involving MDT and a care-coordinator to follow up patient once discharged.

ADULT PSYCHIATRIC DISORDERS

(2) Drug treatments:
- antipsychotics (oral/IM/depot), anticholinergics if extrapyramidal side-effects.
- antidepressants if depression occurs (common after a schizophrenic episode).
- augmentation therapies (add-ons) if antipsychotics alone are not effective: benzodiazepine (short-term sedation only), carbamazepine, antidepressants.

(3) Psychological: CBT for persisting delusions/hallucinations, family therapy for high EE.

(4) Social/rehabilitation: day centres (social skills training, vocational training, education, help with benefits and housing, outings and recreation).

(5) Community care: GP, CMHT, crisis team, assertive outreach team. There has been a shift towards mainly community-based care rather than hospital-based care for those with schizophrenia. Well-organised community follow-up that is integrated with hospital services can increase compliance with medication, reduce the need for hospitalisation and reduce social isolation.

C: Personal and social cost: hospitalisation, strain on relationships, dropping out of education, time off work/job loss.
Suicide: 10% die by suicide, up to 50% attempt suicide.

P: Variable and difficult to predict for any individual.
25% – good (one or two episodes with full recovery).
50% – moderate outcome (undulating course with recovery and relapses and some persistent deficits).
25% – chronic (relapsing, remitting illness with persistent functional disability).
10% die by suicide.

Good prognosis	Poor prognosis
Old age of onset	Young age of onset
Female	Male
Married	Unmarried
No family history	Family history
Sound personality	Personality problems
High IQ	Low IQ
Precipitants	No obvious precipitants
Positive symptoms	Negative symptoms
Treatment compliance	Poor treatment compliance
Low EE	High EE
Acute onset	Insidious onset
Presence of mood component	No mood component

SCHIZOAFFECTIVE DISORDER

There is considerable overlap between schizophrenia and bipolar disorder. Patients are diagnosed with schizoaffective disorder only if they satisfy the criteria for schizophrenia and mood disorder occurring *during the same episode*, but where psychosis is not secondary to mood disturbance.

Treat mood symptoms and schizophrenic symptoms, e.g. lithium and antipsychotics may be used in combination.

Prognosis is better if mood symptoms predominate.

ADULT PSYCHIATRIC DISORDERS

D: Persistent fear and avoidance of social situations that may lead to scrutiny, criticism or embarrassment (e.g. eating, drinking, speaking in public).

A: Unknown. ? Learned behaviour, e.g. previous experience of humiliation/bullying.

A/R: Psychosocial: single, high education and social class, low self-esteem, low mood, general anxiety.

E: F > M. Onset gradual from late puberty: 17–30 years. 8% of phobic disorders.

H: Situational anxiety in social groups: parties, meetings, classrooms.
Fear of being judged negatively by others, resulting in
(1) avoidance behaviour.
(2) anxiety symptoms: blushing, trembling, panic attacks, urgency/fear of micturition.

E: Normal unless exposed to social situation.
A&B: Blushing, shaking, restless, avoids eye contact. Panic.
S: Quiet, shy.
M: Low, fearful.
T: Fear of scrutiny/humiliation. Fear of vomiting/fainting.
C: Normal.
I: Variable. May be good when in normal environment.

M: Graded exposure and desensitisation. Behavioural therapy. Cognitive therapy to address low self-esteem.

C: Isolation.
Depression.
Secondary alcohol abuse/substance abuse.
NB: Dysmorphophobia is increasingly recognised as a separate entity from social phobia. Patients with dysmorphophobia have a persistent irrational fear that some particular part of the body (often the nose or ear) is so grotesquely misshapen as to attract attention in public. Symptoms and avoidances are similar to social phobia, but the focus of the fear is anxiety at others' perceived revulsion caused by the offending body part. Many will seek plastic surgery, although CBT is effective.

D: A group of chronic disorders that are characterised by inappropriate or maladaptive illness behaviours. Patients complain of somatic symptoms and seek medical help. Majority of patients also experience depression and anxiety and the somatisation is usually an expression of personal/social distress. Most patients do not consider themselves psychiatrically ill.

- Somatisation disorder – the patient has a 2-year history of multiple recurrent and frequently changing physical symptoms that cannot be explained by a physical disorder. Chronic form is known as Briquet's syndrome.
- Somatoform pain disorder – the patient has at least a 6-month history of severe distressing pain which cannot be explained by a physiological process.
- Hypochondriacal disorder – the patient has a preoccupation with, and persistent belief in, the presence of one or more serious progressive diseases.

A: Multifactorial. Patients tend to have a low threshold for worrying about symptoms and consulting doctors. Often such attitudes are acquired during childhood when illness behaviour/role is learnt through family/cultural influences. Recent life events also affect illness behaviour, e.g. a family member being diagnosed with an illness. The patient's current psychological status and social situation also determine illness behaviour.

A/R: Anxiety, mood and PDs.
Reinforcement of inappropriate illness behaviour by family, e.g. need patient to maintain sick role and may not be able to tolerate patient's recovery.

E: Point prevalence: 0.5% for severe chronic somatisation.
Commoner in women.
Onset usually before 30 years.

H:
- Multiple recurrent somatic symptoms, e.g. abdominal pain, headache, fatigue, dizziness, pins and needles.
- Multiple investigations/treatments by different specialists.
- Cognitive features: fear, preoccupation with the belief that there is a physical basis to the symptoms.
- Behavioural features: interferes with daily living.

E: MSE – look for features of anxiety, depression, anger or denial.

I: Refusal to accept reassurance leads to multiple investigations for organic aetiology of symptoms.
Exclude organic cause for symptoms. Patients with somatisation disorder have the same risk of developing a new physical disorder as others. All patients must be examined and investigated if they have a new illness.
Differential diagnoses for unusual illness behaviour: dementia, substance misuse, learning disability.
Consider schizophrenia and depressive psychosis (delusions/distorted body image) as differentials for hypochondriacal disorder.

ADULT PSYCHIATRIC DISORDERS

M: (1) Prevention: Doctors can inadvertently reinforce somatisation in many ways. They may fail to acknowledge and treat mood or psychosocial problems. It is important to be clear about negative clinical investigations/findings. Avoid speculative diagnoses, these are often what the patient remembers. Do not arrange investigations/treatment/referrals unless indicated and always explain why. Inappropriate investigations may delay appropriate psychiatric treatment.

(2) General management: Acknowledge the reality of the patient's physical symptoms. Explore the relationship between somatic complaints and possible psychosocial causes. Treat any mood or anxiety disorder. Refer to specialist.

(3) Psychotherapy: To explore underlying problems. Explore the benefits of the sickness role, e.g. release from stress and anxiety (primary gain), increased care from family/sick pay/benefits (secondary gain). Encourage coping strategies and letting go of the inappropriate sick role. Involve family who may be reinforcing the behaviour.

C: Development of chronicity.

P: Often resistant to treatment. If there is no improvement in the first 1 or 2 years, a chronic course is more likely.

ADULT PSYCHIATRIC DISORDERS

D: Persistent fear of a specific object or situation, out of proportion to the threat of the situation. The fear is recognised as excessive, but cannot be reasoned away.

A: Unknown. Many theories on aetiology.
- Conditioning event early in life leads to fear. But most patients cannot recall such an event. Phobias are non-randomly distributed, people more likely to fear natural pre-technological things, e.g. snakes/spiders.
- Learned behaviour, e.g. fear what parents fear.

A/R: • Biological vulnerability to anxiety. Hypervigilant individuals more at risk. Family history increases risk, especially for blood/injury/injection phobia.

E: F = M. 15–20% report phobic symptoms in the community. Onset usually childhood, but may vary.
Blood/injury phobia F > M, 2–3%. Strong link with family history.

H: Core
Fear and avoidance of specific objects/situations.

Four categories of phobias:
animal/insect
situations, e.g. heights, enclosed spaces
blood/injury/injection
natural forces, e.g. lightning, sea

Symptoms of anxiety and panic when exposed to feared stimulus.

Psychological
unpleasant feeling of anticipation and threat
inability to relax
fear of dying/losing control
exaggerated startle response
urge to escape the situation

Biological
sweating
trembling
dry mouth
nausea
difficulty breathing
choking sensation
chill/hot flushes

Most phobias cause tachycardia. But blood/injury phobia causes an initial tachycardia followed by vasovagal bradycardia and hypotension. This may cause nausea and fainting.

E: Normal unless exposed to feared stimulus. When exposed:
A&B: Sweating, restless, panic.
S: Distracted.
M: Fearful.
T: Fear of stimulus out of proportion to actual danger.
C: Poor concentration. Distracted.
I: Good, when away from stimulus they realise it is ridiculous. When stimulus is present, insight is poor.

M: Graduated exposure: prevent avoidance. Avoidance reinforces fears because the patient feels better and safer away from the stimulus.
Flooding: maximum severity exposure.
Modelling: therapist shows that the stimulus is harmless, then the patient tries.
Systematic desensitisation: relaxation therapy paired with exposure.
Drugs: anxiolytics may be used short term only, e.g. diazepam. Not curative.

C: Disruption of normal daily life if the phobic stimulus is something that must be routinely encountered, e.g. crowds, enclosed spaces (lifts etc.).

P: Good. Exposure therapy is often successful. Most phobias do not interfere with normal life if the stimulus can be easily avoided.

A broad term, which may be divided into acute intoxication, abuse and dependence.

D: *Acute intoxication* – transient disturbance of behaviour, cognition or perception after taking a substance.
Abuse – maladaptive and recurrent use of substance leading to significant impairment or distress.
Dependence – may be physical or psychological, or both. Physical dependence may manifest as withdrawal states, increasing tolerance to the substance and increasing use of the substance. Psychological dependence means the patient feels compelled to use the substance, feels out of control and uses despite being aware of adverse consequences of using.

A: Multifactorial, possible neurobiological mechanism. Pre-existing psychiatric conditions, e.g. PDs, ADDH may increase the likelihood of substance misuse.

A/R: Peer pressure, deprivation, availability of substances (and wealth?), iatrogenic factors, e.g. prescription of benzodiazepines/analgesics long term.

E Difficult to assess as people may not be honest about an illegal activity. In the USA 30% of adults admitted to having tried cannabis, 1.5 % had tried heroin.

H&E: Will depend on the substance of choice.

DRUGS AND THE LAW
Maximum penalties
Class A: cocaine, crack, ecstasy, heroin, LSD, magic mushrooms if prepared for use, speed (amphetamines) if prepared for injection.
Possession – 7 years prison and/or a fine.
Supply – life imprisonment and/or a fine.
Class B: cannabis, speed.
Possession – 5 years prison and/or fine.
Supply – 14 years prison and/or fine.
Class C: rohypnol, anabolic steroids, tranquillisers/diazepam.
Possession – 2 years prison and/or fine.
Supply – 5 years prison and/or fine.

I Toxicology screen? Monitor observations closely.

M: If overdose is suspected, specific antidotes may be used, e.g. naltrexone to neutralise opiate effects. General management involves support, rehabilitation, drug treatment centres. Medication needed to reduce withdrawal symptoms. Long-term replacement medication may be needed, e.g. methadone for opiates.
Management of all medical problems, e.g. gangrene from vascular damage, monitoring and treatment of infections, e.g. hepatitis, HIV.
Psychological approaches, e.g. motivational interviewing, group therapy, CBT.

C: Physical complications are given in the table on pp. 86–8. Substance abuse may worsen/precipitate psychological conditions. Social problems – debts, crime, prison (see penalties above). Social isolation.

P: Depends on the substance of misuse. Also depends on social support, motivation.

ADULT PSYCHIATRIC DISORDERS

Physical complications caused by substance misuse

Name	Street names	Class and origin	Effects	Risks
Cannabis	Marijuana, weed, puff, hash, ganja, draw, skunk, shit, blow, pot	Class B. Derived from *Cannabis sativa* plant. Smoked or eaten.	Relaxation, heightened senses. Lethargy.	Affects concentration and short-term memory. Reduced coordination, paranoia, anxiety.
Cocaine	Coke, charlie, snow, C, white	Class A. May be snorted or injected.	Stimulant. Buzz, alert. Confidence. Lasts roughly 30 minutes.	Heart problems, chest pain, convulsions, permanent damage to the inside of the nose. Overdose. Psychosis, post-high depression.
Crack	Rock, wash, stone	Class A. Smokeable form of cocaine.	High, lasts 10 minutes.	Heart problems, addictive. After the high – restless, confused, paranoia, psychosis, depression.
Ecstasy (MDMA)	E, fantasy, rolexes	Class A. Tablets. Often white.	Alert, senses more intense. Energy. Lasts 3–6 hours.	Nausea, sweating, palpitations. Comedown depression. Liver and kidney problems. There have been 60 deaths in the UK.
GHB	Liquid ecstasy, GHB	Colourless liquid in bottles or capsules. Swallowed. No smell but a salty taste. Possession is not illegal, but supply is.	Sedative. Can produce feelings of euphoria. Effects last up to a day.	Sickness, stiff muscles, fits and even collapse. If incorrectly produced, GHB can badly burn the mouth. Very dangerous when mixed with alcohol or other drugs.

Drug	Street names	Form / route	Effects	Risks / dangers
Gases, glues, solvents	Lighter gas refills, tins/ tubes of glue, paints	Sniffed or inhaled.	Dizziness, hallucinations. Lasts 15–45 minutes. Drowsy afterwards.	Instant death. Nausea, vomiting, blackouts, heart problems. Long-term abuse can damage brain, liver and kidneys.
Heroin (diamorphine)	Smack, brown, horse, gear, H, junk, skag, jack	Class A. Opiate analgesic. Brown/white powder. Snorted, smoked or injected. Controlled drug.	Relaxation, drowsiness. Numbness.	Very addictive, tolerance, damage to veins from injecting. Risk of HIV, hepatitis B and/or C from sharing needles.
Ketamine	Special K, K, vitamin K	Tablets/powder snorted. PoM.	Hallucinatory experiences for up to 3 hours.	Numbness, breathing problems and heart failure in excessive doses.
LSD	Acid, tabs, trips	Class A. Tiny squares of paper, often with a picture on one side.	Hallucinogenic. 8–12 hours duration. Effects depend on the user's mood.	Bad trip – intense anxiety, paranoia, feeling out of control. Accidents. Flashbacks. LSD can complicate other mental health problems, such as anxiety, depression and schizophrenia.
Magic mushrooms	'shrooms, mushies	Class A. Main type is liberty cap mushroom. Eaten raw, dried, cooked in food, stewed into tea.	Similar to LSD. Relaxation. Lasts about 4 hours.	Stomach pains, sickness, diarrhoea. Bad trips. Complicate other mental conditions.
Phencyclidine	PCP, angel dust	Usually smoked.	Euphoria, peripheral analgesia.	Impaired consciousness, psychosis.

(Continued)

Physical complications caused by substance misuse (Continued)

Name	Street names	Class and origin	Effects	Risks
Poppers (amyl/butyl nitrate)	Poppers, TNT, liquid gold	Clear/straw-coloured liquid in a small bottle or tube. Vapour is inhaled.	'Head-rush'. Blood vessel dilatation 2–5 minutes.	Headache. Dangerous for people with anaemia, glaucoma, breathing or heart problems. Fatal if swallowed.
Speed (amphetamines)	Speed, uppers, whizz, billy	Class B. Grey or white powder. Snorted, swallowed, injected or smoked. Controlled drug.	Stimulant, increases HR and breathing rate. Energy.	Comedown tiredness and depression, sleep concentration and memory all affected short term. Panic and hallucinations. Psychosis.
Tranquillisers, e.g. diazepam, temazepam	Moggies (mogadon) valium, downers, benzos	Class C. Penalties, PoM.	Calm, relieve tension and anxiety. Drowsiness and forgetfulness.	Accidents. Dangerous if mixed with alcohol. Tolerance and dependence.

In the UK most people drink alcohol. The Royal College of Physicians uses measures of alcohol consumption in relation to whether they are harmful or not.

One unit of alcohol is defined as
10 ml or 8 g of absolute alcohol, approximately:
1/2 pint (284 ml) ordinary strength beer or lager.
1 glass (125 ml) average strength wine.
1 glass (50 ml) fortified wine, e.g. sherry.
1 single measure (25 ml) spirits.

D: Alcohol misuse: consumption of alcohol sufficient to cause physical, psychiatric or social harm.
Levels of alcohol consumption:

- Low risk: men < 21 units/week. Women < 14 units/week.
- Hazardous drinking (intake likely to increase the risk of alcohol-related harm): men 22–50 units/week. Women 15–35 units/week.
- Harmful drinking (this is synonymous with alcohol misuse). A pattern of drinking associated with the development of alcohol-related harm. Men > 50 units/week, women > 35 units/week.

A: Multifactorial. No specific cause. See risk factors below.

A/R: Genetic factors, culture, religion, family history, availability and price of alcohol, males.

E: In the UK, 0.5–1.0% drink harmfully. This number has been increasing over the past decade. Overall, 27% of men, and 13% of women drink over the recommended 'low-risk' level of 21 and 14 units/week. M/F = 2 : 1.

H: See Psychiatric History (Section 1) – taking alcohol history.

E: Physical examination for alcoholic stigmata, and those of chronic liver disease, e.g. palmar erythema, spider naevi, gynaecomastia, peripheral neuropathy, signs of portal hypertension.

MSE will depend on the state of intoxication.

Acute intoxication
A&B: Smell of alcohol, uncoordinated, may have acute injuries.
S: Slurred.
M: Labile, may be excessively happy or sad.
T: Variable.
P: None.
C: Slow, impaired judgement.
I: May be poor.

Acute withdrawal – delirium tremens (usually starts within 48–72 hours after drinking cessation).
A&B: Agitated, tremor, fearful, may have nausea and seizures.
S: Confused.
M: Labile, may be anxious.
T: Delusions.
P: Hallucinations or illusions – usually visual.
C: Confused, poor attention.
I: Poor.

I: Blood alcohol level, LFT, B_{12} and folate, FBC, U&E.

M: Detoxification – support, benzodiazepines to prevent seizures and control hallucinosis. Rehydration and correction of electrolyte disturbances. Vitamin B supplements.

Maintaining abstinence and rehabilitation.
Treat coexisting depression.
Relapse prevention.
Motivational interviewing.
Social network therapy.
Family therapy.
Self-help, e.g. AA.
Physical treatments:
Disulfiram – blocks alcohol dehydrogenase so leads to an unpleasant reaction on drinking. Works best with supervised administration.
Acamprosate – reduces conditioned aspects of drinking and prevents craving-induced relapses.
Naltrexone – opioid antagonist. Reduces reinforcing actions of alcohol, i.e. it reduces the pleasure alcohol gives.

C: Psychological
irritability
anxiety
depression
blackouts
alcoholic hallucinosis
paranoia
morbid jealousy
self-harm
memory loss

Physical
acute intoxication
anorexia
GI upsets (gastritis, ulcers, nausea)
hypertension
cardiac arrhythmias
cardiomyopathy
cirrhosis
hepatitis
jaundice
peripheral neuropathy
dementia
Wernicke–Korsakoff's syndrome (see below)
osteoporosis
foetal alcohol syndrome

Delirium tremens is precipitated by withdrawal. Someone in delirium tremens may experience confusion, hallucinations, ataxia, fits, delusions and anxiety.
Interpersonal: relationship problems, alienation of friends.
Work: loss of job, days off sick, poor performance at work, accidents at work.
Law: drink driving or public disorder offences.
Economic: debts, selling possessions.

Wernicke's encephalopathy – ataxia, nystagmus, ophthalmoplegia and acute confusion. Caused by thiamine deficiency, so responds to administration of thiamine. If untreated may develop into
Korsakoff's psychosis – profound loss of short-term memory. May be associated with a general dementia.

P: Relapsing and remitting. High suicide risk. Depends on support and premorbid personality.

D: Intentional self-inflicted death.
Not all suicide attempts result in actual suicide. It can be difficult to distinguish between those that were intended to be fatal and those that were acts of deliberate self-harm.

A: Psychiatric disorders: depression (hopelessness main predictor); schizophrenia; substance misuse; PD; OCD; AN.
Medical disorders: chronic pain; cancer patients.
Biochemical abnormalities: studies of CSF and brain show reduced 5-HT.
Sociological factors: loss of shared values and reduced social support.

A/R: Age: young men and elderly are at higher risk.
Sex: M > F.
Psychiatric disorders.
Loss events (e.g. bereavement).
Unemployment.
Living alone.
Being single.

E: Accounts for about 1% of all deaths in UK, rates vary between countries.
Highest rates in the elderly, although rates rising in young men.
M/F = 3 : 1.

H: See Psychiatric History section.

E: MSE – may indicate signs of underlying psychiatric disorder.

I: Medical investigations according to the method, e.g. drug levels.

M: (1) Prevention
At individual level:
detection of people at risk of psychiatric disorders
At social level:
reduce ease (e.g. smaller packets of paracetamol)
provide support services (e.g. Samaritans)
reduce stressors (e.g. reduce employment)

(2) Management of attempted suicide
Assess risk and consider admission.
Use section 2 MHA if refusing treatment.
Ensure adequate observation at home/hospital.
Address underlying psychiatric/medical issues.
Follow up by CMHT.

(3) Management of completed suicide
Do not move body until the police arrive.
Inform RMO, manager, police and coroner.
Break bad news to next of kin.

C: Death.

P: 1% of those who have attempted suicide die from suicide within 1 year.

ADULT PSYCHIATRIC DISORDERS

D: Infection with *Treponema pallidum*.

A: Spirochaete infection.

A/R: Usually sexually transmitted.

E: Prevalence decreased following introduction of penicillin, now making a comeback.

H: Need to know sexual history, any contacts also at risk.

Primary – infected painless hard ulcer at site of infection (usually an abrasion).

Secondary – 1–2 months later. Fever, lymphadenopathy, rashes.

Tertiary – rare. 1–5 years after primary infection. Granulomas occur in skin, mucosa, etc.

Quaternary – may lead to meningovascular effects, e.g. delirium, dementia.

8–12 years after primary infection *tabes dorsalis* may occur, in which the patient experiences 'lightning pains'; numb legs, chest and nose; sensory ataxia; flexor plantars; Argyll Robertson pupils.

5–25 years after primary infection general paresis of the insane may occur: personality changes, cognitive changes, dementia, depression or grandiose delusions leading, in extreme cases, to mania or schizophreniform psychosis.

E: Depends on the stage of disease.

I: Cardiolipin antibody detectable in early syphilis. Treponema-specific antibody, e.g. *Treponema pallidum* haemagglutination assay (TPHA).

M: Procaine penicillin. May induce neuropsychiatric improvement even in severe disease.

C: The longer the delay before treatment, the more irreversible changes will occur.

P: Good when detected and treated early.

ADULT PSYCHIATRIC DISORDERS

D: Hepatolenticular degeneration. Copper is deposited in various sites throughout the body, including
cerebrum – dementia
basal ganglia – tremor, rigid akinetic syndrome, choreoathetosis
liver – cirrhosis, jaundice, hepatosplenomegaly
eyes – Kayser–Fleischer rings
bones – osteoporosis, osteoarthritis
kidneys – renal impairment

A: Autosomal recessive, chromosome 13.

A/R: Family history.

E: Rare. 5–30/1 000 000 prevalence.

H: Up to 60% of patients with Wilson's disease have psychiatric symptoms. They may be affective, e.g. depression, behaviour/personality changes, schizophreniform psychosis, cognitive change/dementia.

E: MSE will depend on which psychiatric features the patient presents with.

I: Serum copper is low, caeruloplasmin levels low, hypodensities in basal ganglia seen on CT scanning.

M: Reduce copper levels using dimercaprol. Treat symptoms appropriately.

C: Movement disorders, renal impairment, cirrhosis (see above).

P: Neurological damage is irreversible. Pre-cirrhosis, any liver damage may be reversible. Death is from liver failure, variceal bleeding or infection.

SECTION 4: CHILD PSYCHIATRIC DISORDERS

Rather than 'mental illness', when dealing with children it is often best to think in terms of thoughts, feelings or behaviours which are unusual, e.g. outside the normal age range, and causing significant distress to the child or others.

THE PREVALENCE OF PSYCHIATRIC DISORDERS IN CHILDREN

Two studies are often quoted:

The Isle of Wight study (Rutter, M., Tizard, J. & Whitmore, K. (1970) Education, Health and Behaviour. London: Longman.) found the 1-year prevalence of psychiatric problems in 10–11-year-olds to be around 7%, with a boy/girl = 2 : 1.

Inner London study (Richman, N., Stevenson, E. J. & Graham, P. (1982) Pre-school to School: A Behavioural Study. London: Academic Press.) found the 1-year prevalence of emotional and behavioural problems in pre-school children to be 22%.

RISK FACTORS FOR CHILD/ADOLESCENT MENTAL DISORDERS

The environment
poverty
social deprivation
migration
racism/bullying
peer group pressures
environmental pollution, e.g. lead

The child
low IQ
difficult temperament
specific developmental delay
hearing and communication difficulty
physical illness
low self-esteem
male

Protective factors
positive self-image
adaptable temperament
consistent discipline
adult supervision and encouragement
high IQ or special skill or ability

CHILD PSYCHIATRIC DISORDERS

- Psychiatric disorders can affect normal child development.
- See table for normal developmental milestones/Freud's developmental stages.
- The 'attachment theory' developed by John Bowlby is an important psychological theory that is often taught; it relates to a child's social development.

Age	Social, emotional & behavioural milestones	Freudian stage
0 to 6 months	Smiling, social responsiveness	Oral
6 months to 1 year	Separation anxiety	Oral
	Put food in mouth	
1 to 2 years	Self-help skills, feeding, begin to attain continence, symbolic play with toys, stranger shyness	Anal
3 to 5 years	Attain continence, can dress and undress, can play on their own or alongside others, subsequently learn interactive play	Phallic
Middle childhood: 6 years to puberty	Operational thought – practical and tied to immediate circumstances and specific experiences, increased autonomy and involvement with peer group	Latency
Adolescence	Abstract thought develops – reasoning, concepts, testing hypotheses, relate mostly to peer group	Genital

Freud's theories of child development and identity are very much concerned with the body and with family relations. The identity develops progressively through the phases – oral, anal and phallic.
(1) Oral – mother's breast, satisfied desire, incorporation
(2) Anal – defecation, expulsion/destruction, retention and control
(3) Phallic – awareness of self (genitals), auto-erotic, not separate identity, not recognising 'others'

ATTACHMENT THEORY
- Small babies accept separation from their parents.
- At about 6–7 months of age they start to become attached to a particular individual, known as the attachment figure.
- The attachment figure is usually someone who has had a lot to do with the baby. The attachment is not dependent on the amount of time spent, it is the *intensity* of the social interactions that matters.

NORMAL ATTACHMENT BEHAVIOURS (6 MONTHS TO 3 YEARS)

- When attachment figures leave the room the child will cry, call for them and crawl or toddle after them.
- The child may cling hard when anxious/fearful, tired or in pain.
- Hugging, climbing onto their lap.
- Talking and playing more in their company.
- Using them as a secure base from which to explore.
- All are intensified by anxiety, tiredness or illness, and gradually abate after 3 years of age.
- At the same time as the development of attachment behaviour, a wariness towards strangers is usually developed (about 6 months).

ABNORMALITIES OF ATTACHMENT FORMATION

These categories are derived from Mary Ainsworth's Strange Situation Test (SST). In SST it is the child's behaviour after a period of separation that is important.

Attachment abnormalities	Features	Explanation and prognosis
Absent/ attenuated	• No discrimination between familiar and unfamiliar adults when seeking comfort.	• Unsuitable circumstances, e.g. institutional rearing, emotionally cold/rejecting parent.
	• Relationships may appear intimate, but are superficial and easily broken by separation without separation anxiety.	• Developmental problems, e.g. autistic spectrum disorder.
Avoidant (or anxious–avoidant) attachment	• Child has formed a selective attachment but is insecure.	• May result from the child's natural personality. In this case there is a good prognosis if the child's parents learn to accept this.
	• Child separates easily from parents and plays alone in their absence.	• Can however be a result of harshness, coldness or rejection on the part of the parents. This has poorer prognosis and is associated with future antisocial behaviour.
	• On their return child is indifferent and may even avoid them, or behave aggressively.	
Ambivalent attachment	• The child is ambivalent: chronically clingy and being actively cross with the attachment figure following even brief periods of separation.	• Usually due to a combination of the child's temperament and the parent's state of mind or personality.

(Continues)

CHILD PSYCHIATRIC DISORDERS

(*Continued*)

Attachment abnormalities	Features	Explanation and prognosis
		• These insecure attachments are likely to precede emotional disorder in childhood, particularly school refusal.
Disorganised attachment	• The child displays unusual behaviour on reunion, may even adopt strange postures for long periods, apparently frozen, or compulsively avoiding eye contact.	• This is the pattern most strongly associated with abuse and deprivation.

D: Also known as ADD/H, hyperkinetic disorder. Severe form of long-term overactivity associated with inattention and impulsivity arising during childhood before 6 years of age.

A: **Biological**
genetic (increased risk if family history)
developmental factors
abnormal functioning of inhibitory pathways in parietal and frontal lobe

Psychosocial
poverty
diet (lead, tartrazine)
parental alcohol abuse

A/R: **Comorbidity**
conduct disorder
learning difficulties
antisocial behaviour
depression

E: Prevalence 1–2%.
M/F = 3–4 : 1.

H: Motor overactivity, squirming and fidgeting, inconsiderate of others, difficulty obeying instructions, interrupts others, problems with school work.

E: Development assessment. Full neurological screen.

I: Diagnosed by specialist assessment. Collect information from parents and teachers.

Psychological and educational assessments.

M: (1) Information and support for parents and teachers.
(2) Attend to educational deficits and environmental factors.
(3) Behavioural modification. Educate parents and teachers about appropriate methods – reward good behaviour and discourage reinforcement of problem behaviour.
(4) Exclusion diets.
(5) Drug treatments (under specialist supervision for selected cases only due to risk of side-effects, mainly over 6-year-olds): CNS stimulants to increase frontal activity, e.g. methylphenidate. Side-effects include growth retardation, insomnia, decreased appetite, hypertension, exacerbation of tics.

C: Low IQ/learning difficulties (child does not sit still and learn).
Risk of accidents (due to impulsivity).
Low self-esteem and peer rejection (behaviours upset other children).

P: Usually symptoms reduce by puberty.
Severe cases may persist into adulthood.
Learning difficulties and other comorbidity give a poorer prognosis and may persist.
May develop antisocial personality in adulthood.
Associated risk of drug misuse.

CHILD PSYCHIATRIC DISORDERS

D: Also known as Kanner's syndrome. Autism represents the severe end of a spectrum of pervasive developmental disorders.
Triad of features:
Language and communication difficulties.
Poor/absent social interaction.
Restricted and repetitive behaviour.
This broad category includes Asperger's and Rett's syndrome (see eponymous syndromes in Appendices).

A: Unknown.
No sound evidence for a causal link between MMR vaccine and autism.

A/R: Possible genetic component.
Commoner in social class I and II.
Autism often coexists with learning disability:
40% have IQ < 50, 10% have IQ > 100.
Epilepsy is common in adolescence.

E: Prevalence 2/10 000.
M/F = 4 : 1.

C: Clinical features:
Onset < 36 months. 20% develop autistic features after a period of normal development.
Early symptoms: floppiness, poor eye contact, sluggish feeding.
Social impairments: aloofness, lack of interest in people, unresponsive to social cues, poor eye contact, no capacity to share or understand emotions, failure to develop normal attachment.
Language abnormalities: distorted and delayed speech and language development, echolalia, stilted rate and rhythm of speech, impaired use of gestures and facial expressions.
Stereotyped or ritualised behaviour: hand flapping, rocking, restricted and repetitive behavioural repertoire, insistence on routines, resistance to change, true obsessions/compulsions especially in adolescence.
May have isolated exceptional abilities.

E: MSE
A&B: Ritualised, stereotyped behaviour.
Poor eye contact, aloof.
May attach to unusual items.
S: Delayed speech, echolalia, stilted rate and rhythm of speech, impaired use of gestures and facial expression.
M: Normal.
T: Obsessions and compulsions.
P: None.
C: May have exceptional abilities in certain fields, e.g. maths. Otherwise delayed language development.
I: Poor.

I: Full developmental assessment. Exclude any sensory deficits, e.g. deafness.

M: General principles – early detection, reduce handicap.
Child – treatment of comorbid problems, e.g. ADD/H, epilepsy.
Speech therapy to improve language skills.
Behavioural approach to challenging behaviours.
Parents/family – education. No cure, but aim to reduce handicap.

Support groups, e.g. National Autistic Society.

Family therapy to reduce carer stress.

School – statement of special educational needs.

Special schooling.

Encourage social interaction.

C: Social isolation.

Inability to live independently in the majority.

P: Lifelong disorder.

Better prognosis with early speech acquisition, higher intelligence and signs of diminishing impairments.

CHILD PSYCHIATRIC DISORDERS

D: Disorders characterised by persistent and pervasive antisocial behaviours which violate the basic rights of others and are out of keeping with age-appropriate societal norms/rules. The disorders can be divided into 'socialised' and 'unsocialised'.

'Socialised' – the antisocial behaviour is viewed as normal within the peer group and/or family, and the individual is able to make lasting peer friendships.

'Unsocialised' – the antisocial behaviour is solitary and associated with peer and parental rejection.

A: Exact unknown.
Theories suggest:

Psychosocial issues
family disharmony
parental violence
parenting problems
parental alcoholism
antisocial PD
depression
anxiety

Biological issues
genetic factors
brain damage

A/R: Education problems, e.g. specific reading retardation.
Commoner in those from deprived areas.
Commoner in those in residential care.

E: Prevalence 4%.
M/F = 3 : 1.

H: One episode is not significant enough to make the diagnosis; there must be a 6–12-month history.
Problems reported by parents/teachers/police include:
frequent bad tempers/irritability
disobedience
blaming others for their own mistakes
violence
bullying
forensic problems
inappropriate sexual behaviour

E: MSE.
Physical.
May be difficult, child/adolescent may not engage in conversation.
Their behaviour may be disruptive during the interview.

I: Check for educational difficulties. Developmental assessment.

M: (1) Mild cases may resolve without any treatment. Counselling and practical support may be all that is needed.
(2) Psychotherapies for more severe cases: family, behavioural therapy (focusing on aggression) and group therapies.

(3) Address educational needs with remedial teaching.
(4) Provision of alternative peer group activities.

P: 2/3 continue to have problems into adulthood, many develop antisocial personality disorder. 'Socialised' group have better prognosis.

Elimination disorders – enuresis

D: The involuntary passage of urine in the daytime and/or at night-time, which is abnormal in relation to the child's mental age.

If it occurs solely at night-time, it is called nocturnal enuresis.

A: Multifactorial – see below.

A/R: **Biological**
family history – genetic link
smaller functional bladder volume in those with enuresis
developmental delay

Psychosocial
behavioural problems
family difficulties
stressful life event

E: Prevalence: 10% at 5 years
            5% at 10 years
            1% at 15 years
Boy/girl = 2 : 1.

D: To make the diagnosis the child's chronological and mental age must be at least 5 years.
The voiding must have occurred at least twice in a month in children aged under 7, and at least once a month in children aged 7 years or more.

E: MSE – may be features of anxiety or behavioural disorders.
Physical.

I: To exclude organic pathology, e.g. UTI, structural abnormality of the urinary tract, epilepsy, diabetes.

M: (1) Educate parents about the problem and provide reassurance. Include advice about fluid intake, e.g. limiting bedtime drinks.
(2) Behavioural therapy:
  • Focusing on behaviour modification by rewarding the child for keeping dry, e.g. by use of star charts. The child should not be punished for failing.
  • Other methods include the use of a bell and pad – a buzzer sounds if the pad under the sheet becomes wet, this wakes up the child. The child is then encouraged to go to the toilet and, if old enough, is encouraged to help change the sheet before going back to sleep.
(3) Drug treatments:
  • Synthetic ADH, e.g. desmopressin, applied as a nasal spray.
  • TCA will inhibit enuresis in the short term and may be useful if a child wants to sleep over at a friend's house. They have a toxicity risk and a high relapse rate and therefore should not be used for long-term management.
  • Anticholinergic drugs (e.g. oxybutinin).

C: Problems at school – bullying or isolation, poor self-image.

P: 90% resolve by adolescence.

Elimination disorders – encopresis (non-organic)

D: The child repeatedly passes faeces in places that are inappropriate for the purpose (e.g. the floor), either involuntarily or intentionally.

A: May be due to emotional disturbance.

A/R: As for enuresis.

E: Prevalence 2% boys, 1% girls at 8 years.
For all ages boy/girl = about 3 : 1.

H: Most children are faecally continent by age 4 years – the child must have mental age of over 4 years to make a diagnosis.
There must be reports of at least one encopretic event per month, for the last 6 months.
May reflect anger, emotional disturbance or the child not wanting to be independent.

E: Normal except for anxiety/emotional disturbance.

I: To exclude organic disorders, e.g. overflow secondary to constipation, fissure in anorectum.

M: (1) Explore emotional factors.
(2) Behaviour modification – the child is rewarded for the appropriate passage of faeces, e.g. by a special sticker/star chart.
(3) Psychotherapy and family therapy for managing emotional problems and relationship difficulties between child and parent.
(4) It should be emphasised that the child should NOT be punished if there are problems, and should just be rewarded for getting it right.

P: Almost all cases resolve by adolescence.

CHILD PSYCHIATRIC DISORDERS

D: An impairment of the CNS originating during the developmental period, which presents during early childhood with a below average intellectual performance and reduced ability to acquire life/adaptive skills resulting in social handicap.

Impairment of CNS   **Disability** in learning   **Handicap** in social skills

Type	Mild	Moderate	Severe	Profound
IQ	50–69	35–49	20–34	< 20
Average age of presentation	School age	3 to 5 years of age	Before 2 years of age	Before 2 years of age
Defining features	Limited in school work, but able to live alone and maintain some form of paid employment later in life	Able to do simple work with support, needs guidance or support in daily living	Requires help with daily tasks and capable of only simple speech	Very disabled in all aspects
Achievable mental age	9–12	6–9	3–6	< 3

A: Many cases unknown especially if mild, may be end of normal distribution.
Severe cases may be associated with the following:

Genetic
chromosomal (Down's syndrome, Klinefelter's syndrome)
autosomal dominant (neurofibromatosis, tuberous sclerosis)
autosomal recessive (phenylketonuria)
sex-linked (fragile X)

Structural developmental abnormalities
(hydrocephalus)

Secondary to brain damage
antenatal (infection, toxic, hypoxic, maternal disease)
perinatal (birth asphyxia, intracranial bleed)
postnatal (infection, injury, epilepsy, toxic, metabolic – hypothyroidism and phenylketonuria)

A/R: Social and educational deprivation.
Low parental intellect.

Comorbid conditions
epilepsy
autism
cerebral palsy
hearing impairments
visual impairments

psychiatric disorders
behavioural disorders

E: Overall prevalence 2%.
Of these 80% are mild, 12% are moderate, 8% are severe/profound.

H: Presenting complaints in children:
- delay in usual development (e.g. sitting up, walking, speaking, toilet-training)
- difficulty in managing school work as well as other children
- behavioural problems

Presenting complaints in adolescents:
- difficulties with peers, leading to social isolation
- inappropriate sexual behaviour
- difficulty in making the transition to adulthood

Presenting features in adults:
- difficulties in everyday functioning, require extra support (e.g. cooking and cleaning, filling in forms, handling money)
- problems with normal social development and establishing an independent life in adulthood (e.g. finding work, marriage and child-rearing)

Medical
problems antenatally/perinatally/postnatally
comorbid conditions

Family
inherited disorders
learning disability

E: Physical
head circumference
signs of specific syndromes
neurological examination (especially sight and hearing)

MSE
be flexible in your approach
collateral history from family/carer
screen for comorbid psychiatric problems

Developmental assessment using specialised tools, e.g. Adaptive Behaviour Scales.
Assessment of behaviour and interactions: neuropsychological assessment including IQ testing.

I: Neuroimaging; blood test for chromosomal analysis.

M: (1) Managed by community paediatric team/learning disability services with multi-disciplinary approach to assessment and therapy (e.g. OT, speech therapy, educational support, social support including finance and housing).
(2) Treatment of comorbid medical and psychiatric problems is essential, although unnecessary medication should be avoided (as side-effects are common and underreported).
(3) Give information about support groups.

CHILD PSYCHIATRIC DISORDERS

CHILD PSYCHIATRIC DISORDERS

(4) Give general advice to patient and family:
- Early intervention and continued learning and practising can help, but there are no miracle cures.
- People with learning difficulties are capable of loving relationships and have the same needs as any other person for love, security, play and friendship, together with clear boundaries and limits on behaviour.

Prevention
antenatal screening
genetic testing and counselling
postnatal tests for phenylketonuria and hypothyroidism

C: Patients with learning disability have higher prevalence of psychiatric symptoms than the general population. There can be difficulty in diagnosing psychiatric conditions due to language difficulties and atypical presentations (e.g. schizophrenia may present with simple repetitive hallucinations and persecutory delusions but few first-rank symptoms; in depression, motor and behavioural changes are more key features than verbal expressions of depressed mood).

P: Chronic problem with no cure but the handicap can be modified by social support.

TRUANTING

The child is not at school but not at home either. The parents are usually unaware of the child's whereabouts. Usually happens in groups, and especially in children with conduct disorders. Boys > girls. Associated with learning difficulty, unsupportive home environment.

SCHOOL REFUSAL

This is different from truanting. The child wants to stay at home. It is common around the age of 5 years and 11 years – secondary school age.

Risk factors: vulnerability, parents not able to set boundaries or force children to go to school, children with bereavement issues, ambivalent attachment.

EMOTIONAL DISORDERS

Childhood depression

In children it can be difficult to identify depression because of fluctuating symptoms.

Depression in children is defined as

- low mood (not usually persistent)
- somatisation (see below)
- personality change

As in adults there may be disturbance of sleep and appetite and feelings of low self-esteem. There is a risk of suicide in children as young as 5 years of age! It is not uncommon for a previously well pre-adolescent child to have fleeting suicidal thoughts.

Treatment is with antidepressants.

Somatisation – psychological problems expressed as physical symptoms, e.g. 'tummy ache' in children may often have an emotional cause.

Adolescent depression

15% of adolescents get depressed. Mainly girls. Especially age 14–15 years. Rates stay high until early twenties.

OCD

Rare in early childhood, although isolated compulsions are quite common. It presents as in adults. It may respond to behavioural methods, and also antidepressants, e.g. SRIs.

SLEEP DISORDERS

These are common in children. 20% of children have night-time wakefulness, 3% sleepwalk.

Night terrors – the child sits up terrified and screaming but cannot be woken enough to reassure. Associated with tachycardia and tachypnoea, may be associated with stress. Usually occur at age 4–7 years, especially in children with a positive family history.

CHILD PSYCHIATRIC DISORDERS

CHILD ABUSE

This includes neglect, emotional, physical and sexual abuse.

Risk factors

Unwanted child, mental/physical handicap, young/single parents with their own history of abuse, adverse socio-economic situation.

Signs of abuse

Children who are *physically* abused (non-accidental injury) may have injuries without convincing explanation, bruises of varying ages, delayed presentation of injuries, inappropriate reaction of the parents, injuries inconsistent with the child's stage of development, recurrent injuries. They are at increased risk of emotional and behavioural disorder.

Neglect may present as failure to thrive, inadequate hygiene, poor attachment to the parent, speech and language delays. It may lead to delayed psychological and physical development. Later on they may have persistent low self-esteem, relationship difficulties and PDs.

Emotional abuse includes rejection of the child, malicious criticism, threats and ridicule, scapegoating. These children may develop emotional or conduct disorders. They may exhibit pseudomature behaviour.

Sexual abuse is defined as the involvement of dependent, developmentally immature children and adolescents in sexual activities that they do not fully comprehend, and are unable to give informed consent to. May involve genital exposure, fondling, genital, anal or oral sexual activity or intercourse, including rape.

Risks: poor parental sexual relationship, maternal depression/illness, mother sexually abused in childhood, family disorganised, social isolation, abuser inadequate or aggressive. Abusers usually male, but female abusers are being recognised with increasing frequency.

Presentation: genital trauma or infection, highly sexualised behaviour towards adults or children, pregnancy, unexplained decline in school work or change in behaviour, e.g. fearful reaction to adult men, secondary enuresis.

A full physical examination should be performed by a senior doctor skilled in paediatric examination for child sexual abuse.

Women who were sexually abused are at increased risk of psychiatric disorders in general, and in particular borderline personality disorder, and BN. Men who were sexually abused may become abusers and perpetuate the cycle.

General consequences of abuse: vulnerability to conduct, emotional and developmental disorders, as well as depression and parenting problems in adult life.

Management: enlist specialist help whenever child abuse is suspected. Contact paediatricians, child psychiatrists, social services child protection teams. A full history and examination must be performed. Careful documentation of any injuries, with photographs taken with parental permission. Height, weight and head circumference should be measured and plotted on a centile growth chart. Treat specific injuries.

The child may need immediate protection, admission to hospital may be appropriate (this allows investigations and MDT assessment).

Child Protection Conference will decide whether to place the child's name on the Child Protection Register, whether there should be an application to the court to protect the child, and what follow-up is needed.

SECTION 5: PHYSICAL TREATMENTS

- Always exclude other medical causes that may mimic the underlying disorder.
- Always consider other therapies before prescribing.
- Consider the side-effects, make sure the benefits outweigh the risks.
- Choose the appropriate drug based on side-effect profile, e.g. sedating versus non-sedating.
- Consider possibility of dependence/withdrawal syndromes or toxicity and risk of overdose.
- When a patient complains of any symptom, look at the drug chart; is it iatrogenic?
- Monitor outcome of the therapy (relapse/improvement).
- Always consider drug interactions when combinations of drugs are prescribed.
- Good communication skills are essential to ensure drug compliance.
- Every patient needs to know
  (1) the name of the drug you are prescribing
  (2) the objective of the treatment – to treat the disease/relieve symptoms
  (3) how to take and when to take the medicine
  (4) whether it matters if a dose is missed and what to do about it if anything
  (5) how long the drug is likely to be needed
  (6) how to recognise side-effects and any action that should be taken
  (7) whether there is a need for special monitoring of blood levels of the drug
- This is a lot for the patient to remember – written leaflets are always helpful.
- This is also a lot for the doctor to remember – always refer to the BNF.
- Refer to the BNF for special situations, e.g. prescribing for the elderly, for children, in pregnancy.

PHYSICAL TREATMENTS

PHYSICAL TREATMENTS

EXAMPLES
Citalopram
Fluoxetine
Paroxetine
Sertraline

MECHANISM
Inhibit the reuptake of 5-HT by the presynaptic neurone, so increase the concentration of 5-HT in the synaptic cleft.

INDICATIONS
Depressive illness (treatment and prophylaxis in recurrent episodes)
Anxiety disorders (e.g. GAD, phobic disorders)
BN

SIDE-EFFECTS
Gastrointestinal disturbance (usually transient):
nausea
vomiting
anorexia
weight loss
dry mouth

Sexual:
lower libido
orgasmic difficulties

Neuropsychiatric:
headache
anxiety

CONTRAINDICATIONS
Manic state, use with caution in bipolar disorder

PRESCRIBING NOTES
- Given orally (tablets) usually o.d.
- May take 2 weeks before any effect and 6 weeks for full effect.
- Withdrawal symptoms have been reported (especially with paroxetine).
- Relatively safe in overdose, although some patients have reported increased suicidal ideation initially.

EXAMPLES
Amitriptyline
Imipramine
Lofepramine
Dothiepin

INDICATIONS
Depression
Anxiety disorders (phobic disorders, GAD)
OCD
Chronic pain (e.g. trigeminal neuralgia)
Nocturnal enuresis (imipramine)

SIDE-EFFECTS
Anticholinergic:
dry mouth
blurred vision
constipation
urinary retention
drowsiness

Cardiovascular:
postural hypotension
arrhythmias

Toxicity in overdose:
cardiotoxic
respiratory failure
seizures
convulsions
coma

CONTRAINDICATIONS
Recent MI
Arrhythmias
Mania – use with caution in bipolar disorder

PRESCRIBING NOTES
- Given orally (tablets/solutions) usually o.d. at bedtime.
- May take 2 weeks before any effect and 6 weeks for full effect.
- May cause drowsiness – advise patients to avoid driving.
- Avoid if high suicide risk in outpatient (lofepramine is the safest TCA in overdose).

PHYSICAL TREATMENTS

PHYSICAL TREATMENTS

EXAMPLES
MAOI – irreversible:
Phenelzine
Isocarboxide

RIMA – reversible:
Moclobemide

INDICATIONS
Refractory/atypical depression
Chronic dysthymia

SIDE-EFFECTS
Cardiovascular:
postural hypotension
arrhythmias

Neuropsychiatric:
drowsiness/insomnia
headache

GI:
increased appetite
weight gain

Sexual:
anorgasmia

Hepatic:
hepatotoxic – raised LFT

SERIOUS SIDE-EFFECTS
Hypertensive crisis – due to interactions between MAOIs and tyramine-containing
   compounds (see prescribing notes).
5-HT syndrome – due to interactions between MAOIs and 5-HT-enhancing drugs
   (TCA, SRIs).
NB: Side-effects and interactions are less common with RIMAs.

CONTRAINDICATIONS
Mania – use with caution in bipolar disorder
Hepatic impairment
Cerebrovascular disease
Phaeochromocytoma

PRESCRIBING NOTES
- Given orally (tablets) o.d.
- Patients must carry a card indicating that they are taking MAOIs and must be
  educated and given written information about MAOIs, especially about diet-
  ary requirements.
- Foods to be avoided include cheese, pickled fish, meats, broad beans, yeast
  extracts.
- Patients are advised only to eat food that is fresh and to avoid undercooked
  food.
- Patients are advised to avoid alcohol.
- Other antidepressants should not be prescribed until 2 weeks after cessation
  of MAOIs.

Antipsychotics = Neuroleptics = Major tranquillisers

EXAMPLES

Typicals:
phenothiazines – chlorpromazine, fluphenazine, thioridazine
butyrophenones – haloperidol, droperidol
thioxanthine – flupenthixol
benzamide – sulpiride

Atypicals:
clozapine, olanzapine, risperidone

INDICATIONS

Schizophrenia, psychosis, mania and agitation

MECHANISM

DA receptor blockade. Also block muscarinic, alpha adrenoceptor and histamine receptors. Atypicals block 5-HT and DA receptors.

SIDE-EFFECTS

Typicals	Atypicals
Extrapyramidal: Parkinsonism symptoms, acute dystonia, tardive dyskinesia (long-term) and akathisia.	All have reduced propensity to cause extrapyramidal side-effects. Can all cause diabetes (IGT). All atypicals can cause weight gain and postural hypotension.
Hyperprolactinaemia: impotence, amenorrhoea.	Risperidone: hyperprolactinaemia.
DA receptor blockade.	
Agranulocytosis (rare).	Clozapine: agranulocytosis.
Cholinergic blockade: dry mouth, blurred vision. Alpha adrenoceptor blockade: postural hypotension.	Note: Regular follow-up and leukocyte and differential blood counts required for patients on clozapine. It is restricted to patients registered with the Clozaril Monitoring Service.
Sedation: histamine receptor blockade.	Olanzapine: sedation.
NMS (medical emergency)	NMS less likely.
• Autonomic instability	
• Hyperthermia	
• Raised creatinine phosphokinase	
• Coma	
Other: cholestatic jaundice, photosensitivity, cardiac toxicity – arrhythmias (QT prolongation).	Atypicals should be used with caution in patients with cardiovascular disease (QT prolongation).

PHYSICAL TREATMENTS

PHYSICAL TREATMENTS

PRESCRIBING NOTES

- The typicals are effective in controlling the core positive symptoms of schizophrenia and also for sedation.
- Atypicals have a therapeutic effect on negative symptoms, cognition and mood.
- Withdrawal of treatment requires careful supervision as rebound psychosis can occur when treatment is stopped.
- Pretreatment ECG is required.
- Monitoring of BP, pulse, at regular points throughout treatment.
- May be administered orally or IM. To increase compliance a long-acting depot IM injection can be used (e.g. haloperidol decanoate: one injection every 4 weeks).
- Extrapyramidal side-effects can be reduced with the administration of an antimuscarinic (e.g. procyclidine); note tardive dyskinesia does not improve with such drugs.

Minor tranquillisers = sedatives, also used as hypnotics.

Benzodiazepines and barbiturates. Barbiturates are only prescribed to patients already taking them as severe dependence and tolerance develop readily. Barbiturates are also dangerous in overdose.

Diazepam, nitrazepam – prolonged action.

Temazepam, lorazepam – shorter action.

INDICATIONS

For short-term relief of severe anxiety, insomnia (hypnotic effect), alcohol withdrawal, status epilepticus (diazepam), premedication before minor surgery

MECHANISM

Bind to GABA receptors and potentiate GABA-mediated inhibitory neurotransmission in the CNS.

SIDE-EFFECTS

Drowsiness.

Dependence and tolerance with prolonged use, should only be prescribed for the short term.

Withdrawal syndrome – insomnia, anxiety, loss of appetite and weight, tremor, perspiration and perceptual disturbances. Withdraw in gradual steps.

CONTRAINDICATIONS

Respiratory depression

Severe hepatic impairment (benzodiazepines metabolised in the liver, accumulation of active metabolites can occur)

PRESCRIBING NOTES

- Care with alcohol and other minor tranquillisers as they enhance the sedative effects of benzodiazepines.
- Hangover effect can impair the ability to drive or operate machinery.
- Paradoxical effects – an increase in hostility and aggression can occur in those taking benzodiazepines.
- Flumazenil is a benzodiazepine antagonist that can be given as an antidote in overdose.
- Administered orally (solutions/tablets), IM, IV, p.r. in divided daily doses.

This is the team of people, from various professions, who are responsible for the long-term care of the patient. The advantage of working in this type of team is that the patients' social needs may be addressed. Psychiatric patients depend heavily upon social and non-medical services. MDTs operate on wards, in day hospitals and in the community (CMHT). Distinctions between professional boundaries are more blurred in the CMHT.

MEMBERS OF THE TEAM

Medical: SHO, SpR, lecturer, clinical assistant, associate specialist, consultant.
Non-medical: psychiatric nurse, CPN, social worker, occupational therapist, psychologist, art therapist.
The consultant is the RMO who has legal responsibility for care of patients and who has to sign, e.g. leave forms for sectioned patients.

- Psychiatric nurse – monitoring and observations of patients. May be involved in decision-making about leave arrangements for detained patients. Attends MDT meetings and ward rounds. In an emergency can detain an inpatient under section 5(4) for 6 hours or until a doctor arrives.
- Community psychiatric nurse – member of CMHT. Gives depot injections, assesses mental state, pays regular visits, can be the care-coordinator.
- Social worker – helps manage patients' personal and social problems, e.g. housing, benefits, community groups. May also act as a care-coordinator for a patient under the CPA. Also involved in assessing patients for section under the MHA.
- Occupational therapist – treatment of physical and psychiatric conditions through specific activities in order to help people reach their maximum level of function and independence in all aspects of daily life. Assessment of ADL.
- Art therapist – uses different art forms to gain a reflection of patients' thought and the issues they bring to the art therapy session. May work with individuals or groups. Referral is often by non-medical team members, e.g. OT.
- Clinical psychologist – involved in assessment of patients' suitability for certain types of psychological treatment. May perform intelligence tests, personality assessments. Also assesses patients for civil or forensic purposes. Clinical psychologists also treat patients using cognitive and behavioural therapies, or CBT.
- Patient advocate – not a member of the MDT but helps the patients express their worries/concerns. May attend meetings with the patient to make requests on behalf of the patient. Not involved in making decisions on treatment.

CARE PROGRAMME APPROACH

This is a system of care aimed at addressing patients' psychiatric, psychological and social needs once they are back in the community. It is required for anyone who has had significant contact with psychiatric services, e.g. >3 months inpatient treatment, >3 admissions in the last 18 months, offending patients, following serious suicide attempts, dementia and at risk in their own homes, discharged following detention under the MHA (in which case a section 117 meeting must be held before discharge).

The idea of a CPA is that medical and social services should work together and have regular reviews of the patients' progress. The frequency of review depends on the level of the CPA (standard or enhanced) and the patients' needs.
The care plan is clearly documented. One team member is named care-coordinator for that patient, responsible for coordinating all the service provisions in the community.

Methylphenidate
Dexamphetamine

INDICATIONS

Methylphenidate – hyperkinetic disorder and ADD/H (under specialist supervision only)
Dexamphetamine – refractory ADD/H, narcolepsy

MECHANISM

CNS stimulants: amphetamine (dexamphetamine) and related drugs (methylphenidate). Stimulate areas of the brain (frontal lobes) necessary for focused task-orientated behaviour and channelled attention. The child's behaviour becomes less impulsive.

SIDE-EFFECTS

Decreased appetite with resultant weight loss and possible growth retardation
Rebound hyperactivity
Depression
Insomnia
Headache
GI symptoms (e.g. stomach pain/GI upset)
Theoretically may worsen epilepsy

CONTRAINDICATIONS

Cardiovascular disease
Hyperthyroidism
Predisposition to tics or Tourette's syndrome

PRESCRIBING NOTES

- Very rarely prescribed in children under 6 years.
- Reserve drug treatment for severe cases that have not responded to other interventions.
- High doses may cause slowing of growth in children.
- Drug may be needed for months to years and careful monitoring of height and weight is essential.
- Need to give 4-hourly doses (morning, lunchtime and possibly evening) as drug has a short half-life.

Many different types of therapy – counselling, CBT, psychodynamic psychotherapy, group/family/couples therapy and IPT. They are all 'talking' treatments based on communication between the therapist and client (patient).

COUNSELLING

Brief, focused interventions that are time limited to 6–8 sessions. Effective in primary care settings. As for all therapies it is supportive and non-judgemental, with patients encouraged to express their feelings and discuss their concerns. The aim is to provide emotional support and guidance so the patients can deal with their concerns/crises more effectively.

Indications

Useful for those experiencing bereavement or relationship difficulties/breakdown

Contraindications

Not for those with chronic and serious mental health issues, inadvisable for some personality disordered patients

COGNITIVE–BEHAVIOURAL THERAPY

Derived from two main psychotherapies, behaviour therapy and cognitive therapy. Behaviour therapy is based on the leading theories of Ivan Pavlov (classical conditioning) and B. F. Skinner (operant conditioning) and was developed in the 1950s. Cognitive therapy was developed in the 1960s by Aaron Beck and is closely linked to Albert Ellis' rational emotive therapy. Over the years these therapies have been integrated and are referred to as CBT.

CBT is structured, time limited, problem and goal orientated. Emphasis on problems in here and now. Homework is important and there is emphasis on relapse prevention procedures.

Cognitions: thoughts, beliefs, attitudes or images. CBT aims to alleviate negative thinking and self-defeating behaviour by dealing with distorted cognitions: e.g. a depressed patient may have negative cognitions of himself, a negative view of the world and a negative view of the future (Beck's cognitive triad). Cognitive distortions include all or nothing thinking, catastrophising, disregard of the positive and overgeneralised inferences made from one negative event. CBT aims to identify and challenge underlying assumptions and treat cognitive distortions, replacing these beliefs with alternative and realistic cognitions.

Emotions: somatic symptoms can accompany certain emotions: e.g. a person who is panicking may experience palpitations, sweating, trembling and difficulty breathing.

Behaviour: certain maladaptive behaviours are the result of things we have learned: e.g. an anxious patient may escape or avoid situations/activities that are perceived as threatening. This avoidance results in the reduction of fear, which is a reward, which in itself results in negative reinforcement. The therapy involves identifying the **antecedent** to the behaviour (e.g. panic attack in a crowded place) and the **consequences** of behaviour which are reinforcing the problem (e.g. escaping reduces anxiety).

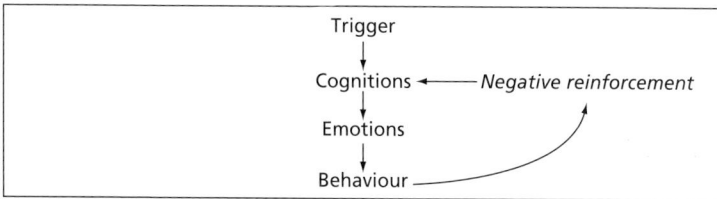

Indications
CBT has been evaluated in randomised controlled trials and has been shown to be as effective as medication in the treatment of:

* depression (mild to moderate)
* eating disorders
* phobic disorders (e.g. agoraphobia, social phobia, specific phobias)
* panic disorder
* GAD
* OCD
* psychosexual problems
* post-traumatic stress disorder

In addition, CBT has been shown to reduce the likelihood of subsequent relapse.

Treatment
The therapist aims to formulate the problem by outlining

* the predisposing factors (e.g. childhood learning experiences)
* the precipitating factors (e.g. life event such as bereavement or stress at work)
* the perpetuating factors (e.g. substance misuse, negative reinforcement from family)

A commonly used behaviour treatment for phobias and obsessions is graded exposure therapy and response prevention. A hierarchy of anxiety-provoking situations is constructed and the patient faces up to these situations in a graded manner. Patients gradually habituate to the anxiety they experience and the anxiety will eventually be easier to tolerate and subside. This is positive reinforcement.

PSYCHODYNAMIC PSYCHOTHERAPY
Based on the psychoanalytical ways of understanding human development as developed by Freud, Jung and Klein. The developmental model stresses that early childhood experiences are crucial in shaping the personality. Treatment involves discussing past experiences and how these have shaped the present situation. Unconscious conflicts are explored and the insight gained aims to change patient defence mechanisms and maladaptive behaviour. The main goals of psychotherapy are symptom relief and personality modification through exploration of the unconscious. There is much emphasis on the relationship between the therapist and patient. Therapies can be offered on an individual, couple, group (hospital ward/day hospital) and therapeutic residential community basis.

Indications
Dissociative conversion disorders, somatoform disorders, psychosexual disorders, certain PDs, chronic dysthymia, recurrent depression, relationship difficulties

Relative contraindications
Antisocial personality disorder, acute psychotic disorders, current depression with high suicide risk.

Treatment
Involves exploring the patient's unconscious through the use of
(1) psychodynamic
- analysis of transference – the attachment of the patient towards the therapist which develops during treatment.
- analysis of counter-transference – the therapist's attitude and feelings towards the patient.

(2) psychoanalytical
- free association – free and uninterrupted flow of words and thoughts.
- dream analysis – interpreted according to the theories of psychoanalysis.

Differences between psychodynamic and psychoanalytical psychotherapies

Type of therapy	Psychodynamic	Psychoanalytical
School of origin	Freudian	Jungian
Frequency + duration	Once weekly, for 1 year	3 times a week, for many years
Location	Patient in a chair	Patient lies on a couch
Major principle of therapy	Principles of transference and counter-transference	Uses free association and dream analysis
NHS/Private	Available on the NHS	Mostly only available privately

GROUP PSYCHOTHERAPY
Problem-sharing in a group setting that develops insight, self-confidence, sensitivity and social skills. There is emphasis on interrelationships between group members facilitated by the therapist. Groups can be ongoing or time limited.

Indications
Eating disorders, alcohol and drug misuse, family problems and as for individual therapy

ART AND MUSIC THERAPY
Non-verbal forms of psychotherapy, with the patient communicating with the therapist via art or music. The therapist encourages free association in the form of art or music with the results interpreted by the therapist as an expression of the unconscious.

INTERPERSONAL THERAPY
Focuses on the connection between onset of symptoms and current interpersonal problems and life events. The focus is on helping the patient's interpersonal/social difficulty to alleviate current symptoms. Usually 10–15 sessions.

Indications
Depression and eating disorders

- A medical procedure used under controlled conditions to treat some major psychiatric disorders including major depressive illness, psychotic depression, mania, puerperal psychosis.
- Generally used when an illness remains unresponsive to other treatments, or the side-effects of drug therapy pose too much of a problem or when an immediate effect would be beneficial.
- The patient is anaesthetised and given a muscle relaxant; seizures are then induced by delivering brief electrical stimuli to the brain via scalp electrodes.
- Patients usually receive a total of 4–12 treatments, given twice weekly.

The exact mechanism is unknown but it is thought to be complex including neurotransmitter release, hormone secretion from the hypothalamus and pituitary, modulation of neuroreceptors, changes in blood–brain barrier permeability.

SPECIAL PREPARATIONS
- ECT is a treatment for which either informed consent or a second opinion is needed (MHA, section 58).
- If the patient is informal, only valid consent is needed. If a patient is being detained under a treatment order but gives valid consent, form 38 must be completed. If a patient is under treatment order and is refusing treatment, form 39 is completed and a second opinion must be sought from an independent consultant appointed by the MHA Commission. Emergency ECT can be given once under section 62 while awaiting a second opinion.
- Patients must have a full pre-operative work-up including any necessary investigations, e.g. ECG, U&E, CXR and assessment by the anaesthetist.

MEMBERS INVOLVED
A nurse, who checks the patient has been nil by mouth and looks after the patient in recovery. An anaesthetist, who gives the muscle relaxant and anaesthetic.
A psychiatrist who administers the treatment.

SIDE-EFFECTS AND COMPLICATIONS
Common side-effects:
confusion
headache
short-term memory impairment

Complications:
cardiovascular problems (arrhythmias)
anaesthetic problems (e.g. laryngospasm/tooth damage)
status epilepticus

SAFETY
- The risk is approximately the same as that for a general anaesthetic.
- (NB: About 10% of those with recurrent depression will commit suicide.)

CONTRAINDICATIONS
- Serious anaesthetic risk
- Raised ICP (as ICP rises during treatment)
- Glaucoma (as intraocular pressure also rises during treatment)
- History of status epilepticus
- Recent MI (< 6 months ago)

DRUG INTERACTIONS

Anti-epileptics and benzodiazepines, e.g. increase seizure threshold.
ECT may result in lithium toxicity (due to dehydration because of being nil by mouth).

INDICATIONS
- BAD (decreases frequency of manic and depressive episodes)
- Augments antidepressants in treatment of refractory depression
- Treatment of borderline and impulsive personality disorder

MECHANISM
Not fully understood.

SIDE-EFFECTS
General:
weight gain
fine tremor
muscle weakness
oedema

GI:
diarrhoea
nausea
vomiting
metallic taste

Renal:
nephrogenic diabetes insipidus (polyuria and polydipsia)
long-term use results in renal scarring and impaired renal function

Endocrine:
hypothyroidism
parathyroid hormone problems – Ca disturbance

Cardiac:
T-wave inversion

Haematological:
leucocytosis

CONTRAINDICATIONS
Pregnancy
Renal disease
Cardiac disease
Addison's disease
Untreated hypothyroidism

PRESCRIBING NOTES
- Prescribed only on specialist advice.
- Narrow therapeutic index and possibility of toxic build-up – therefore should only be prescribed after careful consideration of risk/benefit ratio. (Therapeutic range 0.5–1.0 mmol/L. Increased side-effects above 1.2 mmol/L. Risk of toxic effects above 1.5 mmol/L.)
- Need pretreatment considerations and investigation:
  (1) medication review (NSAIDS and ACE inhibitors interact)
  (2) blood tests – FBC, U&E, thyroid screen, pregnancy test
  (3) ECG
- Need investigations during treatment: check lithium plasma levels twice during first 10 days and then every 3 months; regular monitoring of FBC, U&E and thyroid screen.

- Given orally (tablets/syrup), initially in divided doses until plasma levels stabilise, then o.d.
- Advise patients to consume an adequate fluid intake and to avoid diets which may increase or decrease sodium intake.

Refer to drugs in emergency section for lithium toxicity.

INDICATIONS
Used for bipolar disorder or refractory depression, as well as for all types of epilepsy

MECHANISM
Prevents GABA reuptake so enhances GABA-inhibitory transmission. Reduces concentration of aspartate – an excitatory transmitter. Blocks voltage-gated sodium channels.

SIDE-EFFECTS
Nausea
Vomiting
Weight gain
Rarely hepatic failure
Pancreatitis
Pancytopenia

CONTRAINDICATIONS
Hepatic dysfunction
Porphyria

PRESCRIBING NOTES
- Oral/IV administration.
- LFT should be checked regularly.
- Fewer adverse effects than most anticonvulsants.
- Patients should be given a leaflet about how to recognise haematological/hepatic side-effects.
- Teratogenic.

PHYSICAL TREATMENTS

Mood stabilisers – carbamazepine

INDICATIONS
Used instead of, or in combination with, lithium for bipolar disorder or refractory depression
Also used for treatment of epilepsy and trigeminal neuralgia

MECHANISM
Enhances GABA-mediated inhibitory transmission in the CNS. Reduces electrical excitability of cell membranes by blocking sodium channels.

SIDE-EFFECTS
GI:
diarrhoea
nausea
vomiting
anorexia

Neurological:
dizziness
headache
ataxia
visual disturbance

Haematological:
leucopenia
thrombocytopenia
agranulocytosis
aplastic anaemia

CONTRAINDICATIONS
Atrioventricular conduction abnormalities (unless paced)
History of bone marrow depression
Porphyria

PRESCRIBING NOTES
• Given orally (tablets/solution) often in daily divided doses.
• Pretreatment investigations are needed:
  (1) blood tests – FBC, LFT, U&E, pregnancy test
  (2) ECG
• Regular blood monitoring is required throughout treatment to ensure toxic levels are not reached and to check serum haematological and biochemical levels of the above.

ACUTE DYSTONIC REACTIONS

Due to treatment with antipsychotics such as phenothiazines and haloperidol. Presents with grimacing, facial spasms, especially masseter muscle. May even lead to jaw dislocation, torticollis, limb rigidity and altered behaviour.

Treat with benztropine 2 mg IV bolus, or procyclidine 5 mg IM bolus. Symptoms should improve quickly. Then continue with oral procyclidine 8-hourly if necessary.

CLOZAPINE

Antipsychotic, used in schizophrenia. Has a 3% risk of agranulocytosis. Any patient presenting with fever, sore throat or infection requires FBC to check for neutropenia. If neutropenic, immediately stop clozapine, admit, may need antibiotic and antiviral cover, ITU, G-CSF may be given.

LITHIUM TOXICITY

Lithium is used for treatment of bipolar disorder. However it has a low therapeutic index and so must be regularly monitored. SRIs, antidepressants, anticonvulsants, antipsychotics, diuretics and Ca channel blockers as well as any cause of dehydration can all precipitate toxicity.

Presentation: severe nausea, vomiting, cerebellar signs, confusion, muscular twitching, spasticity, choreiform movements, convulsions, slurred speech, drowsiness, coma, death.

Investigations: serum lithium level, U&E.

Management: stop lithium and give oral fluids in conscious patients, control convulsions with diazepam, haemodialysis for severe poisoning.

MONOAMINE OXIDASE INHIBITORS

May continue to have effect up to 2 weeks after the inhibitors (e.g. phenelzine) are stopped, so during this time no other drugs should be introduced. Acute hypertensive reactions occur following ingestion of tyramine-rich foods, e.g. cheese, yeast extract, red wine. Release of NA causes tachycardia, hypertension and vasoconstriction. May lead to intracerebral or subarachnoid haemorrhage. These hypertensive crises may also be precipitated by sympathomimetics, amphetamines or L-dopa.

NEUROLEPTIC MALIGNANT SYNDROME

A rare complication of antipsychotic treatments. It presents with hyperthermia, fluctuating level of consciousness, muscular rigidity, autonomic dysfunction with pallor, tachycardia, labile BP, sweating and urinary incontinence.

Management: stop antipsychotic. Cardiovascular and respiratory support. Cooling. Bromocriptine may be used but there is no proven effective treatment. NMS usually lasts for 5–7 days after discontinuation of the antipsychotic and may require transfer to ITU. 20% mortality.

PHYSICAL TREATMENTS

PHYSICAL TREATMENTS

THE ACUTELY CONFUSED PATIENT

See Delirium, Dementia and Substance Misuse – Alcohol in Section 3. For Delirium Tremens see Substance Misuse – Alcohol in Section 3.

THE ACUTELY INTOXICATED PATIENT

See Substance Misuse in Section 3.

If the patient is violent – see next page. Try to do a neurological examination and test the blood glucose level.

Comatose patient – medical emergency. Protect airway, and anticipate vomiting. Exclude other metabolic causes of coma, e.g. hypoglycaemia. Exclude head or neck injury. Monitor closely for signs of deterioration, e.g. BP, HR, pupils should be monitored regularly.

THE PATIENT WHO IS NOT EATING OR DRINKING

Management: depressive stupor or schizophrenic catatonia – consider ECT. Remember that the elderly who stop eating and drinking can become moribund very quickly.

Eating disorders: the patient may have to be hospitalised under the MHA and fed on a supervised, high-calorie diet. If that fails, consider IV fluids and feeding by nasogastric tube. See AN and BN for longer-term management.

THE PATIENT WHO HAS TAKEN AN OVERDOSE

Emergency management: ABC, treat shock, consider ventilation if necessary. History from the patient, family or friends.

Try to find out what has been taken, and how long ago. Also try to establish whether alcohol or any other substance was taken.

Physical examination may help to work out what has been taken: e.g. constricted pupils suggest opiates, whereas dilated pupils suggest amphetamines, cocaine or TCA. Respiratory depression may occur with benzodiazepine or opiate toxicity.

Investigations: glucose, FBC, U&E, LFT, INR, ABG, ECG, paracetamol and salicylate levels; urine/serum toxicology.

Management: empty stomach by gastric lavage if it is <1 hour since the drug was taken. DO NOT lavage if corrosives were ingested. Activated charcoal may be used to reduce absorption of some drugs, e.g. salicylate, paracetamol. Give antidote if appropriate.

Poison	Antidote
Benzodiazepine	Flumazenil
Beta blocker	Atropine
Cyanide	Dicobalt edetate
Digoxin	Digoxin-specific antibody fragments
Iron	Desferrioxamine
Oral anticoagulants	IV vitamin K or FFP
Opiates	Naloxone
Paracetamol	N-acetylcysteine

THE SUICIDAL PATIENT/DELIBERATE SELF-HARM

(See also Suicide and Deliberate Self-Harm)

Treat any medical consequences of their actions first.

Keep the patient under close observation and ensure staff are aware of the risk of further self-harm.

Try to assess the patient using the factors below.

Factors suggesting true suicidal intent:

- Careful preparation/premeditation (> 3 hours), e.g. saving up tablets.
- Sorting out their affairs, e.g. will, finances, insurance, etc.
- Taking steps to avoid being interrupted/discovered.
- Violent method of self-harm, e.g. hanging, shooting, high fall.
- Definite, sustained wish to die.
- Hopelessness.

Risk factors for suicide: male, elderly, living alone, separated/divorced, widowed, unemployed/retired, physical/psychiatric illness, alcohol/substance misuse, PD.

If there is a significant risk of future self-harm/suicide, they must be kept in hospital for full psychiatric assessment. Some patients may be discharged with psychiatric outpatient follow-up.

THE VIOLENT AND ABUSIVE PATIENT

Most violent patients presenting to A&E are not mentally ill. They should be referred to the police. Violence associated with psychiatric conditions will be considered here.

Associations/Risk factors: Violence may be more likely if the patient has a past history of violent behaviour, especially if past violence is repeated, sadistic and not accompanied by remorse.

Do not forget to exclude hypoglycaemia, hypoxia and post-ictal confusional states as these may all cause violent behaviour.

At-risk groups: schizophrenia/psychoses, PD, learning disability, post-ictal confusional states, drug overdose, acute brain syndromes (substance intoxication/withdrawal). Young men and those with drug/alcohol misuse are particularly at risk, especially if the precipitants of violence recur repeatedly.

Violence associated with psychiatric illness is relatively uncommon, compared with violence in general.

Ensure safety at all times. Sit between the patient and the door. Make sure other staff know where you are, and that you are aware of how to get help, e.g. 'panic button'. Never turn your back on a patient, especially when leaving the room. Listen to the patient and try not to interrupt.

History: Find out the time and date of any previous incidents, precipitants, amount of social support the patient receives, and whether or not any medications, or other drugs/alcohol are being taken.

Investigations: Blood glucose, toxicology screen, pulse oximetry.

Management: Never attempt to restrain the patient unless sufficient trained staff are available, e.g. three staff trained in 'control and restraint'. Ensure that airway is never compromised at any time. Never try to remove a weapon from a patient, encourage to put it down and then move away from the area together. Patient may need to be sedated for safety. Both antipsychotics, e.g. haloperidol, and sedatives, e.g. diazepam, may be used. Use diazepam emulsion to give diazepam IV (titrate against effects). It may not be possible to take a history from the patient. If a relative is present, try to get a collateral history. Violence may be more likely if the patient has a past history of violent behaviour.

Complications: Injury to patient, staff or other patients: criminal acts should result in prosecution.

Prognosis: Depends on reducing precipitants and improving support.

APPENDICES

- A group of psychiatric disorders with diverse characteristics, which were first described in a particular population or culture. They remain closely associated with these populations. However, they do not currently fit into any particular Western classification system of psychiatric disorders.
- We should remember that some of the disorders that are categorised in classification systems such as ICD-10 are actually specific to Western culture, e.g. AN, and therefore may be considered culture-bound syndromes by other cultures.
- The table below gives some examples.

Disorder	Associated places	Features
Amok	Indonesia; Malaysia	• Unprovoked episode of destructive behaviour including suicide and homicide, followed by amnesia (the patient has no recollection of the event) and fatigue. • May be precipitated by intense anxiety, hostility or humiliation.
Dhat	India	• Male patients complain of a white discharge in the urine which they attribute to being semen. This is accompanied by features of anxiety. • May be precipitated by excess coitus, urinary disorders, dietary problems.
Koro	South-East Asia; South China; India	• Acute panic or anxiety reaction involving fear of genital retraction and subsequent death. • Precipitants are thought to include interpersonal conflicts, illness, excess coitus.
Latah	Indonesia; Malaysia	• An exaggerated response to fright or trauma characterised by echolalia, echopraxia or trance-like states.
Nervios	Central and South America	• Chronic episode of extreme sorrow or anxiety combined with somatic complaints such as headache, muscle pains, nausea, insomnia. • May be part of a grief reaction or as a reaction to stress, low-self esteem and emotional distress.
Taijin Kyofusho	Japan	• Anxiety or phobic disorder. Problems include fear of social contacts, self-consciousness and fear of contracting disease. Somatic symptoms such as headaches and insomnia. • Sufferers are often intelligent and may be perfectionists.

APPENDICES

Asperger's syndrome
A pervasive developmental disorder characterised by abnormalities of social interaction and a restricted, stereotyped, repetitive range of interests/activities. It is part of the autistic spectrum, however, unlike autism, there is no general retardation in language or cognitive development, and IQ is in the normal range.

Briquet's syndrome
A chronic severe disorder in which patients present with bodily symptoms that are unexplained by any medical condition. Sufferers are often female and may suffer from anxiety, depression, panic disorder and PDs.

Capgras's syndrome
A type of delusional misidentification. (See also Frégoli.) Psychotic state characterised by a delusion in which the patient believes a relative or close friend has been replaced by a double.

Cotard's syndrome
Psychotic state characterised by a nihilistic delusion in which the patients believe their body parts do not exist or that they are already dead.

Couvade's syndrome
A somatoform-like disorder where the patient experiences symptoms resembling those of pregnancy including abdominal swelling, spasms, nausea and vomiting in expectant fathers. Anxiety and aching pains are also common.

Da Costa's syndrome
A somatoform disorder (also known as cardiac neurosis) whereby symptoms of autonomic arousal related to the heart and cardiovascular system are attributed by the patient to be due to a physical disorder.

De Clérambault's syndrome
Also known as erotomania. A psychotic state (classically in women, increasingly seen in men) characterised by unfounded and delusional beliefs that someone else, usually of a higher social or professional status, is in love with them. The patient may make inappropriate advances to the person and become angry when rejected. Some stalkers suffer from this.

Down's syndrome
A genetic disorder – trisomy of chromosome 21. It is the most common cause of learning disabilities.

Ekbom's syndrome
Also known as delusional parasitosis. A psychotic state characterised by delusions in which the patient believes that insects are colonising the body, particularly the eyes and the skin. The patient may present at dermatology clinics or to infectious diseases physicians, requesting deinfestation.

Folie à deux
Also known as induced psychosis. A delusional belief that is shared by two or more people who are closely related emotionally and only one of whom has other psychotic features. The pair are often isolated either in terms of distance or by cultural or language barriers. The psychotic individual tends to be more intelligent and better educated, and often has a dominating influence over the other person.

Frégoli's syndrome
A type of delusional misidentification. (See also Capgras.) Psychotic state characterised by the presence of a delusion in which the patients believe that their persecutor has taken on a different appearance, e.g. they may believe that their persecutor is masquerading as their doctor or nurse.

Ganser's syndrome
A type of dissociative disorder in which the patient gives approximate, absurd and often inconsistent answers to simple questions, e.g. when asked how many legs a cow has (the Ganser question) they may reply seven. Other dissociative symptoms may be present.

Gélineau's syndrome
Also known as narcolepsy. A disorder in which the patient, usually a young man, suffers from irresistible attacks of inappropriate sleep along with symptoms of cataplexy, sleep paralysis and hallucinations.

Gerstmann's syndrome
A name given to a combination of symptoms – agraphia, finger agnosia, acalculia, and confusion of left and right sides – that may occur when the patient has a dominant parietal lobe lesion.

Gilles de la Tourette's syndrome
A disorder in which the patient suffers uncontrollable motor and vocal tics, including blinking, nodding, stuttering, coprolalia, palilalia, echolalia and echopraxia.

Kanner's syndrome
Also known as childhood autism. It is a pervasive developmental disorder resulting in language difficulties combined with poor social interaction and restricted repetitive behaviours, usually associated with learning disability.

Landau–Kleffner syndrome
Also known as acquired aphasia with epilepsy. A disorder associated with epilepsy particularly affecting the temporal lobe in which there is a severe loss of expressive and receptive language skills over a period of a few months. The level of non-verbal intelligence and hearing ability are not affected.

Munchausen's syndrome
A type of factitious disorder, which is characterised by deliberately feigned symptoms, these may be physical, e.g. chest pain, or psychiatric, e.g. hallucinations. The patients present many times to hospital clinics and casualty departments. They often give false addresses and have no regular GP. When discovered they usually appear angry and discharge themselves from hospital against medical advice.

There is a variation of this disorder known as Munchausen's syndrome by proxy, in which a mother or carer fakes the illnesses of the child.

Othello syndrome
A psychotic state characterised by the presence of a delusion in which the patient (usually male) believes that his spouse is being unfaithful. The patient may go to great lengths to try to produce evidence of the infidelity and is at risk of being violent and committing homicide.

Wernicke–Korsakoff's syndrome
These are two different phenomena that can occur together and result from thiamine deficiency, Korsakoff's syndrome may follow Wernicke's encephalopathy. Those affected often suffer from alcoholism.

Korsakoff's syndrome is a reduced ability to acquire new memories (i.e. a loss of short-term memory). The patient confabulates to fill in the gaps.

Wernicke's encephalopathy is a disorder of acute onset (hours to days) resulting in global confusion (apathy, disorientation and disturbed memory), eye disturbance (nystagmus and ophthalmoplegia) and ataxia.

Forensic psychiatrists comprise 4.4% of all psychiatrists in the UK.

Forensic psychiatry deals with the interface between psychiatry and the law. It has two broad subdivisions: criminal and civil.

Criminal: the assessment of mentally ill people facing criminal charges. It involves giving evidence about psychiatric defences, recommendations to the courts about disposal.

Civil: civil law (family law, competence, etc.), civil litigation (claims for damages etc.).

Forensic psychiatry is also involved when considering treatment in secure settings. This includes assessment and treatment of non-offenders with difficult or dangerous behaviour, and assessment of dangerousness.

Forensic psychiatrists deal with two systems:

Criminal justice system	Mental health care system
Police stations	Inpatient:
Magistrates courts	Open wards
Crown courts	Local locked (low-security) wards
Remand prisons	Medium-security hospitals
Sentenced prisons	High-security hospitals
	Outpatient:
	CMHT
	Forensic Outreach Services

The number of psychiatric beds has fallen sharply since 1990. This means that there is a shortage of hospital beds, resulting in short admissions and premature discharge. Of patients who are discharged, 12.9% are readmitted within 90 days. As the number of psychiatric beds has fallen, so the number of people held in prison has risen.

THE DIFFERENT TYPES OF PSYCHIATRIC INPATIENT CARE
Open wards
These are the admission wards in local psychiatric hospitals. In Inner London, 60% of these patients are detained. There has been an increase in the levels of disturbance in these wards over the past 20 years, because less severely ill patients are now cared for in the community. There is extreme pressure on beds, and rapid patient turnover.

Local locked (low-security) wards
These have locked doors, higher staffing than in open wards, intensive care function, relatively rapid turnover (weeks or months), more civil orders. These wards are often located in general psychiatric hospitals.

Medium-security hospitals
There are approximately 1400 beds in NHS units. These are supplemented by 400 beds in the independent sector. There are 1–3 units in each health region. They have air-locked entrances, locked internal doors, unbreakable windows, secure garden areas, high nurse–patient ratios, control and restraint training, and minimal perimeter security. Average length of stay: up to 2 years.

High-security hospitals

This type of inpatient care is for those who present a grave and immediate danger to the public. In March 1999 there were 1340 inpatients. Three such hospitals are:

- Broadmoor, Berkshire
- Rampton, Lincolnshire
- Ashworth, Merseyside

They have perimeter and extensive interior physical security. Average length of stay is 8 years.

OTHER ELEMENTS TO FORENSIC SERVICES

Psychiatric services to prisons
Psychiatric MDT/CMHT
Outpatient clinics
Specialist services, e.g. sex offenders, anger management
Probation liaison services
Court and police station diversion schemes
Expert reports for solicitors, courts, CPS, etc.

HOW IS A PATIENT SECTIONED UNDER THE MENTAL HEALTH ACT?

The MHA (1983) has four categories of mental disorder: mental illness, mental impairment, mental retardation and psychopathic disorder. For a short-term section the presence of a mental disorder is sufficient. For longer-term sections the category of mental illness mentioned above should be specified. Note that mental impairment alone does not qualify for detention; it must be associated with aggressive behaviour or irresponsible conduct.

The MHA does not define mental illness: it is left as a matter for clinical judgement.

The MHA does not regard drug addictions, promiscuity, immoral conduct and sexual deviancy as evidence of mental illness. It therefore cannot be used for compulsory treatment for one of these unless the patient has an additional problem that fits into one of the four categories of mental illness.

ARRANGING A MENTAL HEALTH ACT ASSESSMENT

An MHA assessment is activated by telephoning the duty ASW or the duty psychiatrist. They will need information on the following: name, date of birth, address, reason for the assessment, previous history, including name of any care-coordinator, next of kin and past history of violence or self-harm. Enough information must be given so that the ASW can decide if there is a possibility of an admission under the MHA, and that the full assessment process is warranted.

The ASW then takes responsibility for coordinating the assessment, bringing relevant papers and ensuring the process complies with the law. The assessment should ideally be carried out within 5 days.

If the patient is suffering from the short-term effect of drugs, alcohol or sedative medication, discussion should take place about deferring the assessment until a more productive interview can take place.

During the assessment the patient is interviewed to determine whether

(1) there is evidence of mental illness.
(2) there is a risk to the person or others around them.

If there is either of these then:

- Are there any alternatives to admission, e.g. giving medication at home, crisis services, day hospitals, CPN visits?
- Will the patient consent to informal admission?

If admission is decided, the level of security should be determined by the admitting team. The psychiatrist makes arrangements for a bed and the ASW organises the transport. The ASW usually accompanies the patient.

Civil admission orders
Patient must be suffering from a mental health disorder of 'a nature or degree which warrants the detention of the patient in hospital'.

Section	Sectioned by	Duration
4	1 doctor and ASW	72 hours (to assess for section 2)
2	2 doctors (1 psychiatrist) and ASW	28 days assessment
3	2 doctors (1 psychiatrist) and ASW	6 months treatment

Court/Home Office admission orders

Section	Sectioned by	Duration
35	1 doctor	Assessment, pre-sentence – 28 days
37	2 doctors (1 psychiatrist)	Post-sentence – 6 months
41 restriction order	Crown Court Judge	Crown Court Judge or Home Secretary's permission required prior to discharge

Patient already in hospital

Section	Sectioned by	Duration
5 (2)	Doctor in charge	72 hours detention for section 2 assessment
5 (4)	Nurse	Can detain for 6 hours if no doctor available

Guardianship

7 & 8	Guardian	Can require patient to live in a certain place and attend appointments etc.
25A	Psychiatrist	Supervised discharge

Consent to treatment

Section	Purpose
58	Treatment requiring consent or second opinion
59	Treatment requiring consent and second opinion
62	Urgent; can start ECT where condition life-threatening

Other powers

Section 136 – Police can detain person in safety for up to 72 hours.

Section 135 – Magistrate can warrant allowing entry to premises to search for and remove patients thought to need urgent attention.

Section 117 – After-care responsibilities of health and social services, when someone has been detained for treatment.

LEGAL TERMS AND CRIMINAL PROCEEDINGS

What is muteness?

A person refuses to speak and offer a plea to a charge. The jury has to decide whether the defendant is mute by choice or because of a mental illness. If it is decided that it is by choice, the trial proceeds with a 'not guilty' plea.

What is meant by 'fitness to plead'?

Whether or not the defendant is capable of comprehending the trial process and evidence sufficiently to plead and to make a proper defence. It concerns the person's mental state at the time of the trial. The defendant must have the capacity to

(1) understand the nature of the charge.
(2) understand the difference between guilty and not-guilty.
(3) instruct a solicitor.
(4) understand the evidence.
(5) follow the proceedings in court sufficiently as to challenge a juror.

Fitness is decided by the jury after hearing psychiatric evidence. If the person is deemed unfit, a second jury is brought in for a 'trial of the facts'. A range of outcomes is available to the court, from absolute discharge to hospital detention under the equivalent of a restriction order. Being unfit to plead is associated with a severe mental illness or mental impairment.

What is the 'insanity' defence?

'Not guilty by reason of insanity.' This is a retrospective diagnosis of the person's mental state at the time of committing the offence. McNaughton criteria must be met: 'At the time of committing the act, the party accused was labouring under such a defect of reason, from disease of the mind, as not to know the nature or the quality of the act he was doing, or if he did know it, that he did not know that what he was doing was wrong.'

What is 'diminished responsibility'?

This reduces the charge of murder to manslaughter. Homicide Act 1957: 'When a person kills he shall not be convicted of murder if he was suffering from such an abnormality of mind as substantially impaired his mental responsibility for his acts.'

The range of outcomes is from probation to life imprisonment.

What is infanticide?

This is when a woman, by any wilful act or omission, causes the death of her child under the age of 12 months if, at the time of the act or omission, the balance of her mind was disturbed by reason of not having recovered from the effect of giving birth, or of lactation she is deemed to have committed infanticide. This allows the court to pass any sentence.

What is meant by automatism?

'The state of a person who, though capable of action, is not conscious of what he is doing...i.e. unconscious involuntary action.'

The behaviour must be due to disease of the mind. This is a legal rather than medical definition. The person is called 'insane' if the behaviour is likely to recur, e.g. sleepwalking, tumour, epilepsy. Sentence is left to the discretion of the judge.

'Sane' automatisms are once-only events, e.g. concussion, hypoglycaemia, beesting, dissociative states. The outcome in sane automatism is acquittal.

ETHICAL ISSUES IN PSYCHIATRY

Respect for autonomy, i.e. deliberated self-rule. As far as possible, the patients should be allowed to make decisions regarding their treatments. See below for situations when this is not possible.

Beneficence and non-maleficence – there should be a net benefit from treatment, with as little harm as possible.

Justice, e.g. fair distribution of resources, respect for people's rights, and legal justice (i.e. respect for morally acceptable laws).

Consent

For consent to be valid, the patient must be given relevant, specific information relating to the nature and purpose of the procedure/treatment and to its risks/benefits, be able to understand what is proposed in the way of treatment, and give consent voluntarily.

A patient must be legally competent to consent to, or refuse, treatment. Competence relates to the specific procedure, e.g. a psychotic patient can still consent to have the appendix removed.

Competent persons are those who have reached 16 years of age, and have the capacity to make treatment decisions on their own behalf.

Capacity is the ability of the patient to comprehend and retain treatment information, believe that information, and weigh it to arrive at a decision.

Competent adults have the right to refuse medical treatment, even if this refusal results in death or permanent injury. The doctor must confirm that the patient has the necessary capacity to refuse treatment.

If a patient is not capable of consenting to treatment, the doctor can only treat lawfully under the doctrine of necessity, i.e. the treatment is in the patient's best interests. The next of kin is not able to give or withhold consent on behalf of the patient, i.e. there is no proxy consent for an adult.

Research on mentally ill patients

The practice of research on human subjects requires specific ethical criteria to be met:

(1) There should be a reasonable expectation that the research will produce an increase in knowledge that is directly or indirectly relevant to patient care.
(2) There should be no practical possibility that the same increase in knowledge could be achieved other than by working with patients.
(3) The potential benefits (to the research subject or others) arising from the expected increase in knowledge should be of sufficient importance to outweigh any risks of harm inherent in the research.
(4) Patients should give valid consent to their participation in research.

Psychiatric research requires application of these principles. However, there are some difficulties:

(1) The knowledge base in psychiatry is less well established than in other medical disciplines, so there is more debate between experts about the likely extent of any increase in knowledge from research.
(2) There is less scope for research on animal models in psychiatry.
(3) There are practical problems such as how to measure benefits/risks and outcomes.
(4) Psychiatric illnesses may interfere with the patient's ability to make and carry out decisions, so they are more vulnerable to covert pressure.

SLE – depression or psychosis.

Hyperthyroidism/Hypothyroidism – anxiety or depression.

Elevated cortisol – depression or mania.

Low cortisol – depression, lethargy.

Hyperparathyroidism – depression, apathy, memory impairment.

Phaeochromocytoma – anxiety, palpitations, mimics anxiety disorders.

B_{12} deficiency – dementia, depression, psychosis.

Thiamine deficiency – see Alcohol Misuse and Psychiatric Emergencies for details of Wernicke's and Korsakoff's syndromes.

Any infection of brain substance (encephalitis) or meninges (meningitis) may cause temporary psychiatric symptoms.

PSYCHIATRIC SEQUELAE OF HEAD INJURY
Aetiological factors
Background:

premorbid personality

family psychiatric history

personal psychiatric history

Organic:

amount of brain damage

location of brain damage

epilepsy

Current:

emotional

insecure environment

compensation

Classification
- Neuroses (post-concussion syndrome (10–20% after severe injury)) – mild depressive symptoms, irritability, lethargy, fatigue, somatic symptoms, hypochondriasis, loss of libido.
- Personality change – may occur even without brain damage. Premorbid personality traits may become exaggerated. With brain damage there may be personality changes or dementia associated with frontal lobe damage.
- Psychoses – may occur following head injury, especially psychotic depression or schizophreniform disorders.
- Cognitive impairment – commoner with long post-traumatic amnesia, penetrating injuries, haemorrhage, infection, increasing age, and left parietal/temporal lobe damage in particular. Recovery of cognitive function may continue for more than 10 years.

PSYCHIATRIC ASPECTS OF SLEEP DISORDERS
Disorders of excessive somnolence: narcolepsy, Kleine–Levin syndrome, idiopathic hypersomnia.

Disorders of initiating and maintaining sleep: sleep apnoea/Pickwickian syndrome, alcohol, hypnotic withdrawal, restless legs syndrome, neuroses, depression.

Disorders associated with sleep or partial arousal: nightmares, night terrors, somnambulism (sleepwalking).

Disorders of sleep/wake cycle, i.e. jet lag.

Abnormal perceptions: abnormalities in the way information from the outside world is sensed and processed, i.e. hallucinations, illusions.

Acute intoxication: changes in physiological and psychological responses due to the administration of a psychoactive substance.

Affect: the behaviour a person exhibits, which reflects the underlying mood/emotions.

Agitation: feelings of tension combined with excessive physical activity.

Agnosia: patient cannot interpret sensations properly although there is nothing wrong with the sensory organs.

Agranulocytosis: acute deficiency of neutrophils. Neutropaenia is a reduced number of neutrophils.

Ambivalence: simultaneous opposing impulses towards something.

Amenorrhoea: the absence or stopping of menstrual periods.

Amnesia: inability to recall past experiences/events.

Anhedonia: no longer finding pleasure in previously enjoyable activities. Not being able to enjoy anything.

Anorexia: loss of appetite.

Attention: the ability to focus on a specific activity.

Blunted affect: reduced expression of emotion.

BMI (Body Mass Index): calculated as weight (kg)/height (m)^2. It is a measure of body weight in comparison to the general population. Normal BMI is in the range 20–25.

Cathartic colon: atonic colon due to chronic laxative abuse.

Choreiform movements: jerky involuntary movements, particularly affecting the head, face or limbs. Usually due to a disease of the basal ganglia, but may result from drugs used to treat Parkinson's disease, or withdrawal of phenothiazines. They are characteristic of Huntington's disease.

Circumstantiality: a form of thought disorder characterised by speech in which the main point of what is being communicated is lost in a sea of unnecessary trivial details.

Clouding of consciousness: the patient is drowsy and does not respond completely to stimuli. There is disturbance of attention, concentration, memory, orientation and thinking.

Cognition: mental processes by which knowledge is acquired and acted on. Includes perception, reasoning, creativity and problem-solving.

Compulsion: repetitive stereotyped act performed, despite knowing it is senseless, in order to reduce anxiety, and in response to obsessional thoughts.

Concentration: the ability to maintain attention.

Concrete thinking: lack of abstract thought. Normal in children. Occurs in adults with schizophrenia or organic brain disease, e.g. 'People in glass houses shouldn't throw stones – because they would break the windows.'

Conditioning event: establishment of a new behaviour by modifying the associations between a stimulus and a response.

Confabulation: gaps in memory are unconsciously filled with false memories/explanations.

Coprolalia: the repetitive speaking of obscene words.

Counter-transference: the therapist's emotions and attitudes to the patient.

Defence mechanism: mental mechanisms that protect the consciousness from the affects, ideas and desires of the unconscious.

Déjà vu: illusion of familiarity of a situation.

Delirium: disorder of consciousness in which the patient is acutely disorientated, restless and confused. May also experience hallucinations and anxiety.

Delusion: a firm, fixed belief which is held unshakeably and is out of keeping with the patient's cultural/social background. (See Psychiatric History and Mental State Examination for more details.)

Delusional perception: new and delusional significance is attached to a familiar real perception without any logical reason.

Dementia: chronic, progressive, global organic impairment of intellectual functioning without change in consciousness.

Denial: refusal to accept that something is true. Sometimes a psychological reaction to bad news, used as a defence mechanism.

Dependence: psychological and/or physical effect of habitual use of a drug/substance. Leads to compulsion to keep taking the drug. In physical dependence there are withdrawal symptoms if the drug is stopped. Psychological dependence means the person feels the need to keep taking it for well-being, but there are no physical withdrawal effects.

Depersonalisation: an unpleasant sensation where the person feels unreal or strangely altered, or feels that the mind has become separated from the body. Mild forms can occur in normal individuals under stress.

Derealisation: a feeling of unreality in which the environment is experienced as unreal and as flat, dull or strange. Can be very frightening. Often occurs at the same time as depersonalisation.

Displacement: defence mechanism in which thoughts and feelings about one person or object are transferred onto another.

Diurnal mood variation: variation in mood during the course of the day.

Dizygotic twins: twins formed from fertilisation of two eggs. Share half the same genes. They are no more alike than siblings.

DSM-IV: (*Diagnostic and Statistical Manual of Mental Disorders*, 4th edn.) published by the American Psychiatric Association and used in the USA (see ICD-10).

Dysphasia: disorder of language as a result of cortical damage affecting the generation and content of speech. Aphasia is a complete absence of speech due to cortical damage.

Dysthymia: chronic low mood not meeting requirements for a depressive episode.

Dystonia: postural disorder caused by disease of the basal ganglia. Spasms in the muscles of the shoulders, neck, trunk and limbs.

Echolalia: pathological repetition of the words spoken by another person.

Echopraxia: pathological imitation of the actions of another person.

EEG (electroencephalogram): measures the electrical activity of the brain. Reflects the state of the patient's brain and level of consciousness.

Ego: part of the mental apparatus that is present at the interface of the perceptual and internal demand systems. It controls voluntary thoughts and actions and, at an unconscious level, defence mechanisms.

Egodystonic: unpleasant/uncomfortable.

Egomania: pathological preoccupation with oneself.

Elated mood: more cheerful than normal. Not necessarily pathological.

Encopresis: incontinence of faeces.

Enuresis: involuntary passage of urine.

Erotomania: delusion that the individual is loved by some person, often a person of some importance.

Euphoria: exaggerated feeling of well-being. It is pathological.

Euthymia: normal mood.

Flight of ideas: speech consists of a stream of accelerated thoughts with abrupt changes from topic to topic. The connections between topics may be chance relationships, verbal associations, e.g. alliteration, but can usually be followed (unlike Knight's move thinking). Associated with pressure of speech.

Formication: a somatic hallucination in which insects are felt to be crawling on/under skin.

Free association: articulation of all thoughts that come to mind.

Habituation training: training to decrease reaction and sensitivity to a fearful stimulus.

Hallucination: sensory experience in the absence of a stimulus. May be auditory, visual, olfactory, gustatory, tactile. Occurs in normal people when falling asleep (hypnagogic) and waking (hypnopompic). A pseudohallucination is where the patient knows that the hallucination is coming from inside the mind. Visual/tactile hallucinations may imply an organic problem. Auditory hallucinations suggest psychosis.

Hallucinosis: hallucinations occurring in clear consciousness, e.g. in alcoholic hallucinosis.

Hyperacusis: increased sensitivity to sounds.

Hyperaesthesia: sensations appear increased.

Hypoaesthesia: sensations appear decreased.

Hypochondriasis: fear of having a serious illness, in the absence of any real organic pathology.

Hypoglycaemia: low blood glucose.

Hypokalaemia: abnormally low blood potassium.

Hypoxia: deficiency of oxygen in the tissues.

Iatrogenic: condition that has resulted from medical treatment/intervention.

ICD-10: (10th revision of the *International Classification of Diseases*) published by the World Health Organization, Geneva, 1992. Used in Europe (see DSM-IV).

Id: an unconscious part of the mental apparatus which is partly made up of inherited instincts and partly by acquired, but repressed, components.

Ideas of reference: patients feel that other people look at or talk about them, or that TV/media refers to them.

Illusion: false perception due to misinterpretation of a stimulus arising from an object.

Inappropriate affect: an affect that is inappropriate for the circumstances, e.g. giggling when talking about the death of a loved one.

Initial insomnia: difficulty falling asleep when first going to bed. Middle insomnia is waking in the middle of the night. Early morning insomnia (also known as late insomnia) is waking in the early hours and being unable to go back to sleep.

Insight: degree of correct understanding the patient has of the condition and its cause, as well as the willingness to accept treatment.

Jamais vu: illusion of failure to recognise a familiar situation.

Jargon aphasia: incoherent, meaningless, neologistic speech.

Knight's move thinking: odd, tangential associations between ideas leading to disruptions in speech, which means that the connections between topics cannot be followed (unlike flight of ideas).

Labile affect: affect repeatedly and rapidly shifts, e.g. anger to sadness.

Lanugo hair: fine hair covering the body and limbs of human foetus. Also used to describe fine body hair that grows in AN.

Life events: psychologically stressful events in life (such as bereavement, divorce, moving house, changing jobs, etc.), which may trigger onset/relapse of psychiatric conditions.

Logoclonia: the last syllable of the last word is repeated.

Loosening of associations: the connections between a patient's sentences are difficult to follow.

MDT (Multi-disciplinary team): the whole team of health professionals taking care of a patient. May include psychiatrist, psychologist, CPN, ASW, OT, speech and language therapists, etc.

Monomania: pathological preoccupation with a single object.

Monozygotic twins: twins resulting from fertilisation of a single egg. Identical – they have identical genes.

Mood: pervasive and sustained emotion that colours the person's perception of the world.

Mutism: total loss of speech.

Negativism: motiveless resistance to commands and attempts to be moved.

Neologism: a new word invented by the patient, usually with a personal meaning.

Neurosis: a psychiatric disorder in which the patient has insight into the illness, and can distinguish between subjective experiences and reality.

Obsession: intrusive or unwanted thought, image or idea, which enters the patient's consciousness despite attempts to suppress it.

Organic disorder: disorder due to change of structure of an organ or tissue, i.e. a physical disorder.

Overvalued idea: unreasonable and sustained intense preoccupation maintained with less than delusional intensity.

Palilalia: a word is repeated with increasing frequency.

Parasuicide: an act of self-harm in which the motive is not a wish to die. It is different from attempted suicide.

Passivity phenomenon: delusional belief that an external force is controlling aspects of the self, e.g. thoughts, impulses, actions.

Perseveration: mental operations, speech and behaviour carried on beyond the point at which they are appropriate.

Phaeochromocytoma: small tumour of the adrenal medulla. Causes increased adrenaline and NA, increased BP and HR, and palpitations.

Post-ictal: after a fit/seizure.

Posturing: an inappropriate or bizarre bodily posture adopted continuously over a long period.

Poverty of speech: very reduced speech.

Pressure of speech, pressure of thought: speech is very fast, as though there are too many ideas to verbalise all at one time. Occurs in mania and psychosis.

Prodrome: a symptom indicating the onset of a disease, e.g. strange feelings/ aura before an epileptic fit, periods of depression before first schizophrenic episode.

Projection: a defence mechanism in which repressed thoughts and wishes are attributed to other people or objects.

Prosopagnosia: inability to recognise faces.

Pseudodementia: clinically similar to dementia, but has a non-organic cause, e.g. depression, hypothyroidism.

Pseudohallucination: a form of imagery arising in the subjective mind, lacking the substantiality of normal perceptions.

Psychoactive substance: substance which acts on the brain to alter mood/state of arousal.

Psychomotor: muscular and mental activity. Muscular activities are affected by cerebral disturbance.

Psychomotor agitation: excess overactivity and restlessness, e.g. in agitated depression.

Psychomotor retardation: reduced muscular and mental activity. May occur in treatment with neuroleptics, but is characteristic of depression.

Psychosis: being out of touch with reality but with clear consciousness. Characterised by the presence of delusions and hallucinations.

Puerperal: relating to childbirth or the period that immediately follows it.

Regression: a defence mechanism in which there is a return to an earlier stage of development.

Repression: defence mechanism in which there is pushing away of unacceptable ideas and wishes, which remain in the unconscious.

Rumination: an obsessional type of thinking in which the same thoughts or themes are experienced repetitively, to the exclusion of other mental activity.

Section: refers to sections of the MHA, loosely used to denote an order for compulsory admission to a psychiatric hospital.

Serotonin: (also known as 5-hydroxytryptamine (5-HT)) a neurotransmitter thought to be reduced in depression. Also involved in sleep regulation.

Sick role behaviour: activity by individuals who consider themselves ill.

Skin conductance: a measure of the activity of the autonomic nervous system.

Somatic symptoms: relating to the body rather than the mind.

Somatic passivity: delusional belief that one is a passive recipient of bodily sensations or movements from an external agency.

Stereotypy: repeated regular fixed pattern of movement or speech which is not goal-directed.

Superego: partly conscious and partly unconscious derivative of the ego that exercises self-judgement and holds ethical and moralistic values.

Tardive dyskinesia: involuntary chewing or grimacing movements due to long-term treatment with neuroleptics.

Thought blocking: a sudden interruption in the train of thought occurs, leaving a blank after which what was being said cannot be recalled.

Thought broadcast: the feeling/belief that thoughts are audible to others or are being broadcast on television/radio.

Thought insertion: feeling/belief that thoughts are being put into the mind, or are being altered by an external force.

Thought withdrawal: the feeling that thoughts/ideas are being taken out of the mind by an external force.

Tics: repeated irregular movements involving a particular group of muscles.

Torticollis: the head is held constantly to one side.

Transference: the unconscious process in which emotions and attitudes experienced in childhood are transferred to the therapist.

Word salad: the speech is an incoherent and incomprehensible mix of words and phrases.